Family Approaches to Major Psychiatric Disorders

CLINICAL INSIGHTS

Family Approaches to Major Psychiatric Disorders

Edited by
MELVIN R. LANSKY, M.D.

Adjunct Professor of Psychiatry, UCLA Medical School; Chief, Family Treatment Program, Brentwood VA Medical Center; and Faculty, Los Angeles Psychoanalytic Institute

AMERICAN PSYCHIATRIC PRESS, INC.
Washington, D.C.

Note: The authors have worked to ensure that all information in this book concerning drug dosages, schedules, and routes of administration is accurate at the time of publication and consistent with standards set by the U.S. Food and Drug Administration and the general medical community. As medical research and practice advance, however, therapeutic standards may change. For this reason and because human and mechanical errors sometimes occur, we recommend that readers follow the advice of a physician directly involved in their care or the care of a member of their family.

Manufactured in the U.S.A.

The paper used in this publication meets the minimum requirements of American National Standard for Information Sciences—Permanence of Paper for Printed Library Materials, ANSI Z39.48-1984. ∞™

Library of Congress Cataloging in Publication Data

Main entry under title:

Family approaches to major psychiatric disorders.

(Clinical insights)
Collection of papers expanded from a symposium, "Family therapy and major psychopathology," presented at the 1984 Annual Meeting of the American Psychiatric Association in Los Angeles.
Includes bibliographies.
1. Family psychotherapy. 2. Mental illness—Treatment.
3. Terminally ill—Mental health. I. Lansky, Melvin R. II. American Psychiatric Association. Meeting (137th: 1984: Los Angeles, Calif.) III. Series.
[DNLM: 1. Family Therapy—congresses. 2. Mental Disorders—therapy—congresses. WM 430.5.F2 1977 1984]
RC488.5.F324 1985 616.89′156 85-18494
ISBN 0-88048-088-2 (soft: alk. paper)

Contents

Contributors

Marvin L. Adland, M.D.
Training and Supervising Analyst, Washington Psychoanalytic Institute; Clinical Professor of Psychiatry, Georgetown University School of Medicine, Washington, D.C.; and Consultant, National Institute of Mental Health and National Institute on Alcohol Abuse and Alcoholism, Rockville, Maryland

Carol R. Bley, M.S.W.
Program Director and Chief Social Worker, Family Treatment Program, Brentwood VA Medical Center, Los Angeles

Louis Cozolino, Ph.D.
Department of Psychology, UCLA, Los Angeles

Yolande B. Davenport, M.S.W.
Chief, Unit of Family Studies, Laboratory of Clinical Studies, National Institute on Alcohol Abuse and Alcoholism, Rockville, Maryland

Edward Kaufman, M.D.
Professor in Residence and Director, Psychiatric Education, Department of Psychiatry and Human Behavior, University of California, Irvine

Melvin R. Lansky, M.D.
Adjunct Professor of Psychiatry, UCLA Medical School; Chief, Family Treatment Program, Brentwood VA Medical Center, Los Angeles; and Faculty, Los Angeles Psychoanalytic Institute

Barnet Malin, M.D.
Staff Psychiatrist, Brentwood VA Medical Center; Assistant Professor of Psychiatry in Residence, UCLA Medical School; and Clinical Associate, Los Angeles Psychoanalytic Institute

Geneva G. McVey, R.N., C.
Head Nurse, Family Treatment Program, Brentwood VA Medical Center, Los Angeles

DAVID K. WELLISCH, Ph.D.
Associate Professor of Medical Psychology and Department of Psychiatry, UCLA School of Medicine, Los Angeles

KATHRYN L. WEST, Ph.D.
Clinical Psychologist, Family Treatment Program, Brentwood VA Medical Center, Los Angeles; and Assistant Clinical Professor, Departments of Psychology, Psychiatry, and Biobehavioral Sciences, UCLA, Los Angeles

Introduction

This collection of papers is expanded from a symposium, "Family Therapy and Major Psychopathology," presented at the 1984 Annual Meeting of the American Psychiatric Association in Los Angeles. Although the 1984 panelists were also contributors to *Family Therapy and Major Psychopathology*, published in 1981 (1), the panel was more than a mere update of the earlier book. That volume was an attempt to apply family therapy to the major disorders in psychiatry, many of which family therapists of the 1960s and 1970s had ignored. Family therapy was treated as a modality separate from other modalities. Many contributors to the book warned about maneuvers of the family therapist that reacted to or fostered splitting off of treatment modalities and subsequent lack of treatment integration. However, except for the last two chapters, the book fell short of providing an integrative view of treatment. The present book focuses on the importance of an integrated approach for maximally effective treatment, and on the role of family therapy in working toward such an approach.

The emphasis of the 1981 book was on family treatment strategies in major illness, and aimed at avoiding treatment failure. Such treatment ffailure often results from a lack of overall integration in treatment and from a splitting off of the treatment (often pharmacologic) of biologic or constitutional deficits from the therapy of conflict (i.e., psychotherapy). The disarray that results often reflects uncertainty in the mind of the therapist, either about the nature of the basic disorder or about the role of dynamics. If, for example, dynamic factors leading to a schizophrenic patient's drug refusal are not explored by the therapist, dysfunctional interpersonal relationships in the patient's current life circumstances are likely to continue or even escalate and thus threaten the entire treatment effort. If the patient's family is not seen, or if the family is seen by a therapist who is isolated from the person giving medications to the patient, the treatment program is not integrated. Such splitting or one-sidedness usually detracts from the overall effectiveness of the pharmacotherapy. Furthermore, clinical difficulties that arise cannot be properly handled by either medication or psychotherapy in isolation. Likewise, if a patient with manic-depressive psychosis is treated entirely by biological methods, the impact of interpersonal psychological events that trigger severe mood swings (for example, narcissistic wounding and separations) is seldom appreciated by the physician, and the overall course suffers. Or if the physician responds to a person with impulse-ridden character pathology with medication but without an understanding of the relationship of narcissistic wounding to the psychopathology, long-lasting control over the symptoms is unlikely. Splitting between treatment of deficit and that of conflict occurs at the cost of the success of treatment.

I will highlight the evolution of the family therapy movement over the last third of the century in order to provide added perspective on the significance of integrative family treatment.

THE EVOLUTION OF FAMILY THERAPY

Family therapy began in the early 1950s with the observation by many early investigators that schizophrenic patients had a striking preponderance of relatives who seemed either peculiar or outright psychotic. Some of these investigators began the study of the family of the schizophrenic, including many psychoanalysts: Murray Bowen, Don Jackson, Lyman Wynne, Theodore Lidz, and Stephen Fleck. At that time, under the sway of advances in ego-psychology, psychoanalysis was dominated by its interest in the adaptive point of view. Aided by a sensitivity to the adaptive significance of symptoms of all sorts, the investigators hypothesized that schizophrenia might to some extent be an adaptation to a disorganizing and confusing familial environment on which the present or future schizophrenic was dependent and from which he or she could not escape. Hopes were high for gaining an understanding of the possible role of intrafamilial factors not only in the genesis of schizophrenic disorders but even in a new treatment method—family therapy—that might effect a reversal of schizophrenic pathology.

The early investigators described interpersonal and transactional phenomena never before appreciated by clinicians. They evolved concepts and descriptive terms for phenomena that Kraepelinian and psychoanalytic psychopathology could not so vividly describe. The Palo Alto group—Bateson, Jackson, Weakland, and Haley (2) —extrapolated from Bateson's observations on animal play and posited the double bind, an intense disorganizing pattern of communication in which the person at risk for schizophrenia receives conflicting injunctions at different logical levels, together with an injunction not to leave the field. Lyman Wynne and his colleagues (3) described pseudo-mutuality in the family relations of schizophrenics and the "rubber fence"—the sudden rebound back into the family by the pathologic patient who appeared to be leaving the emotional field. Murray Bowen (4) hospitalized entire families containing a schizophrenic member, and in his study of them he developed an intergenerational schema that saw children with low "differentiation of self" trapped in "triangling"—or serving to stabilize—immature parental marriages. Such absorption of parental immaturity comes at the cost of further failure of differentiation of self. According to Bowen, these persons were destined to marry equally undifferentiated offspring of similar marriages and their own offspring would be required to "triangle" even more immature marriages. By this declension into ego fusion, the theory argued, a schizophrenic is eventually formed. Lidz and Fleck (5) and their colleagues at Yale described cross-generational coalitions, marital "schism" and "skew," and "masking" of gross defects in at least one parent, in their well-studied sample.

Each of these groups made major conceptual innovations in studying family processes and describing pathological phenomena. They agreed on concepts such as ego fusion, blurred boundaries, cross-generational coalitions, difficulty in individuating, and ambiguous, bizarre communication patterns. Nonetheless, no convincing evidence has been put forward to support the view that the basic difficulty in schizophrenia arises as an adaptation to the family, or as the result of malignant family processes. Furthermore, family therapy has not succeeded in reversing the basic disease process in schizophrenia.

These early studies have not been fruitless. Discoveries have emerged which have been of lasting value for an understanding of psychopathology in families, for the practice of family therapy, and for psychotherapy in general. These include methods of conceptualizing ego boundaries, coalitions, collusions, and communication, and the corresponding therapist's skills of metacommunicating—communicating about communication. In addition, a great deal of light has been shed on the malignant effects of "scapegoating"—that is, defining (by word or by deed) part of a family system as defective, and highlighting and even provoking those defects in the service of protecting other family members, or the therapist, from exposure as inadequate.

The early investigations of the family shaped the course of the next several decades of family therapy. For example, conceptualization of the identified patient as the family scapegoat (6), and awareness of the effects of reinforcement of the role of the scapegoat by means of the label "sick," have inclined family therapists away from a medical model, with its role assignments of "healer" and "defective." The fact that family therapy has often been done by nonmedical professionals has augmented the antipathy to the medical model in family therapy circles—an antipathy that has prevailed until quite recently. As a new generation of family therapists emerged, they were motivated to treat families in which the identified patient was less severely disturbed than a schizophrenic and whose treatment was more likely to be successful. As the profession developed, all of these factors combined to remove family therapists from the hospital setting and from the most seriously disturbed patients.

The splitting off of family therapy from general psychiatry occurred almost simultaneously with the advent of new and effective pharmacologic agents for many psychiatric disorders, beginning with chlorpromazine and reserpine in the early 1950s, and soon including tricyclics, MAOIs, and lithium carbonate. Indeed, pronounced splitting characterized the entire psychiatric field, as both psychotherapists and psychopharmacologists hoped for cures or at least substantial remissions by their methodology alone. Family therapy, now dominated by antimedical, antipsychoanalytic, and antidisease biases, kept the focus off the hospitalized patient and often off serious consideration of individual psychopathology altogether. General psychiatry, under the sway of the new pharmacologic treatment possibilities, took a neo-Kraepelinian turn, with emphasis on disease entities, course of illness, and medication response that could be measured for specific biologic interventions.

Such a split was justifiable while the new disciplines isolated themselves in order to develop and perfect their unique methodologies. As the disciplines of systems-oriented family therapy and biological psychiatry evolved over the next two decades, however, it became clear that the isolation of psychotherapeutic and psychopharmacologic therapies had left the overall treatment of the most disturbed patients underdeveloped. The "adolescence" of family therapy in the 1960s and 1970s was dominated by a surface idealization, hero worship, separatism, and tendencies toward radical denial of both illness and professional expertise. But as with any healthy adolescence, underneath this bluster was a genuine advance of skill and a consolidation of identity that has enabled family therapists to move forward to a more integrative stage, and to return to the most disturbed patients, who most need their skills. This consolidation of identity in the family therapy movement has recently been combined with an increasingly more usable base of knowledge gleaned from the field of biologic psychiatry (7) and from the newer concepts in psychoanalysis, such as Kohut's ideas (8). The resulting integration includes, for example, the relation of narcissistic vulnerability to the symptom disorders of which alcoholism is perhaps the paradigm; the use of knowledge of family systems to modify favorably the course of major psychotic illness; and the use of an understanding of systems to integrate the family system with the overall health care system in organic disorders (9).

INTEGRATIVE FAMILY THERAPY

The ensuing chapters have enough in common to justify calling them efforts in integrative family therapy. Such therapy assumes that there are diseases leaving chronic deficits and posing treatment obstacles that cannot be definitively cured or reversed. Integrative therapy concerns itself with amelioration in the clinical course of such illnesses, not necessarily with cure. Although etiologies may be ascertained and cures attained in some cases, neither etiologic assumptions nor cure are central therapeutic preoccupations. The therapist, then, cannot assume that one therapy alone, either biologic or psychotherapeutic, provides complete and definitive reversal of pathology. Problems posed by major illnesses are both chronic and complex; the therapist must see them not simply in the isolation of the consulting room but in terms of symptoms, personality, family and ethnic system, and the interaction of these with health care systems.

Family therapy is indicated in the majority of such cases but is rarely the only treatment modality used. Hence, integration is necessary between the individual and the family and between the family and health care systems. The therapist regarding the individual with major pathology, somatic or psychiatric, should keep in mind the enduring deficits posed by the illness and the effects of those deficits on the patient's personality system and family system. Likewise, the therapist is called upon to deal with the interface between the family dealing with illness in its midst and the systems that administer health care. The latter, as is the case with any social system, are organized not only around performing their tasks but also around meeting their defensive needs—for example, avoiding being overwhelmed, exposed as inadequate, or overburdened beyond the capacity of their resources. Each system must be considered dynamically if the patient's and family's care is to proceed optimally and if difficulties are to be understood and overcome.

Within this conceptualization, "dynamics" must be viewed in a system-oriented framework. This framework does not assume that the origin of the patient's basic difficulties is interpersonal, nor that definite cure of them can result from psychotherapeutic interventions—for example, by abreaction or correction of fantasied distortions. Rather, real and enduring deficits are recognized as impinging on both individuals in the family and on the family system, so that avoidance of unpleasure (anxiety, guilt, shame) or maintenance of narcissistic equilibrium (avoidance of humiliation or of exposure of inadequacy or lack of control) often takes precedence over realistic collaboration to correct or minimize the morbidity due to illness. The family evokes defenses to avoid being overwhelmed and to maintain narcissistic equilibrium in the face of illness that threatens that family. Such situational protectiveness often buttresses pathological defenses of the family that predate the illness. These combine to form a heightened defensiveness that often shows up in unproductive relationships with the health care systems. Such defensive and collusive familial relationships can evoke strong reactions from health care systems, which often see them as stubborn, provocative, or even self-sabotaging. In turn, the health care systems become defensive, fearing that they themselves will be overwhelmed by unmanageable demands or be exposed as inadequate or out of control. The results of such constellations, if unscrutinized and not minimized, are splitting of what should be a collaborative team into factions organized around their own defensive needs. The therapist in such an emotional climate may find in himself (or in others) omnipotence or competition with other treatment units; reactivity—for example, anger or inappropriate protectiveness that feeds additional anxiety into the larger system; overregulation; and distancing or outright rejection of the family or patient.

A therapist with this systems view of dynamics recognizes that enormous demands are made on him in the treatment situation.

He or she must be a virtuoso psychotherapist, with knowledge of individual and family dynamics in cases ranging from routine to highly complex and upsetting. The latter occur where splitting and projective identification in collusive systems inject great anxiety into the various parts of the system, provoking further collusion, excessive reactivity, or rejection. The integrative family therapist must deal with these phenomena in disorders that cannot be presumed to have an interpersonal origin. Accordingly, he or she must have a fairly substantial knowledge of disease entities and of the specific treatment systems, hospital and otherwise, that provide assessment, care, and rehabilitation for these disease entities.

The requirements are so encompassing that the therapist's personal development cannot be expected to proceed evenly in all areas. In all probability the development of the practitioner of integrative family therapy will proceed in a biphasic pattern similar to the evolution of the field of family therapy itself. The therapist's training begins with the basics of general psychotherapy and requires a period of omnipotent absorption in family therapy that is split off from other considerations and stays self-contained until the therapist's identity is established. After the therapist's identity is consolidated, he or she will be able to relinquish the omnipotence and sense of self-sufficiency that are only appropriate for the relatively minor disorders treatable by family therapy alone. Only after that maturity has been reached can the integrative aspects of the family therapist develop. It is this capacity to integrate oneself into a complex set of systems and still remain a disciplined therapist that allows the therapist to deal effectively with the patient, the family system, and the systems of health care delivery that intermesh in the treatment of major pathology.

The six chapters that follow highlight integrative family treatment strategies in three areas: the relation of symptom disorders to family system and personality; the psychoses; and family systems medicine—the confluence of family systems thinking and somatic medical treatment.

The chapter on the narcissistically vulnerable marriage and its masks draws from psychoanalytic views of narcissistic and borderline patients to describe the relation of symptom to family system in such disorders. Many families containing one highly symptomatic member, no matter what the etiology of the disorder, have a high degree of narcissistic vulnerability in the disturbed person or in other members, which poses obstacles to what might otherwise be considered a straightforward, symptomatic treatment of the disturbances. Such vulnerable persons have extreme susceptibility to personality disorganization. They have an exquisite sensitivity to shame when this propensity to disorganize becomes exposed or when the collusive relationships that keep them from disorganizing get either uncomfortably close or too far away. Many chaotic-appearing symptoms are found to have a complex distance-regulating effect in the family—that is, to re-equilibrate a highly sensitive system of fragile intimates into a stably unstable coalition (10).

Edward Kaufman's chapter on alcoholism surveys some of the vast amount that has been learned in the last two decades about alcoholism: its demographics, its response to treatment, and its intrafamilial and ethnic context. Considered as a single diagnostic entity only a few decades ago, alcoholism is now recognized as a very complex disorder, colored greatly by familial, ethnic, and personality variables. Kaufman considers the role of ethnic factors and gender on the world of the excessive drinker and on the treatment setting. Although simplified, these portraits underscore the necessity of understanding not only the family context but also the cultural and ethnic givens of the patient's world and how they affect the treatment. Kaufman discusses structural and psychodynamic psychotherapy, and self-help organizations (Alcoholics Anonymous, Al-Anon, and Alateen), essential components in the treatment of most alcoholics that must be integrated into overall treatment if it is to be effective. He shows an exemplary ability to forego the kind of therapeutic omnipotence that insists that treatment be contained in the consulting room and done according to the therapist's specifications. The result of the integrative capacity and flexibility that Kaufman advocates has been a vastly increased capacity to see alcoholics and their families as treatable.

Yolande Davenport and Marvin Adland's chapter on manic-depressive couples, the first of two contributions on the psychoses, summarizes their years of treating such patients in the research-oriented context of the National Institute of Mental Health. Davenport and Adland's clinical attempts are integrative in two major ways: First, they are able to conceptualize a role for development and psychodynamics in a disorder with unquestioned genetic and constitutional "biologic" features. This sophisticated view of psychodynamics does not presume a unique etiologic role for developmental difficulties, nor does it posit psychotherapy as a unifactoral treatment. Rather, the biologic vulnerabilities of the person at risk for manic-depressive illness are seen as contributing to the developmental delays and arrests that become part of the psychopathology, and the psychotherapy is seen as clarifying vulnerabilities and how they are handled in the marriage, regardless of how those vulnerabilities arose. Second, Davenport and Adland are able to integrate therapy of individual and marital units in a treatment that is both dynamic and supportive of limitations posed by the disorder.

The chapter by Kathryn West and her colleagues at the Family Treatment Program at the Brentwood Veterans Administration Medical Center describes a psychoeducational component that has been integrated into the family treatment of schizophrenic patients on an inpatient program in which families are seen in every case. The chapter emphasizes the educational component rather than the entire integrated therapy package.

Although schizophrenia is a chronic illness that is not cured by treatment interventions, the human environment affects the course of the illness profoundly. A clear relation has been demonstrated between sustained exposure to pathological family transactions and a worse-than-expectable course for schizophrenic illness (11). Such pathological families are characterized by what has been called high negative expressed emotion (EE). High EE comprises a clingingness that keeps other family members in unusually close contact with the schizophrenic patient without a realistic appraisal of the illness, and a high proportion of transactions in which the patient is severely criticized without acknowledgment of the possible role of illness in his or her behavior. A change in the patient's exposure to such criticism, either by removal from the family or by a change in the nature of the transactions, often ameliorates the course of illness, changing it to one similar to that in families low in negative expressed emotion.

Psychoeducational approaches are often conceived of as direct attempts to modify high EE family transactions by conveying an understanding of both illness and the malignant effects of criticism on the patient. The extent to which such pathological transactions are actually modified by brief programs is uncertain at present, but psychoeducational approaches need not be justified solely by the surmise that they are likely to modify pathological transactions. By providing information and problem-solving skills, such programs add to the family's repertoire of ways of coping with the illness.

A lengthy appendix gives actual transcripts from the presentations given to families. Although the emphasis is on one component of a treatment program, this contribution is integrative. The effect of a kindly, collaborative team effort at enlightening patient and family has enormous dynamic significance. The patient and family are welcomed as collaborators, and their ignorance and struggles are empathically anticipated and taken seriously. Educational material is presented in ways that relieve the family's worries that they will be blamed for the patient's illness or be saddled with unending demands for support and resources. Permission and encouragement to enjoy life independently from the schizophrenic patient is implied or explicit.

The entire psychoeducational enterprise raises serious questions about what had heretofore been the common practice of *not* telling psychiatric patients and their families either what is wrong with them or what is known about the illness. The ability to so enlighten patients and their families has proceeded *pari passu* with the increase in knowledge of these disorders and their impact. It might be said that in integrative treatment the field has evolved and matured to the point where failure to educate would be as cruel and incompetent as it would be in disorders such as hypertension and diabetes mellitus!

The final two chapters are concerned with the family treatment of serious somatic pathology in the context of the entire health care system. The emergence of family therapy as a major element in the treatment of somatic illness has gained enough momentum in recent years to warrant the founding of a significant new journal, *Family Systems Medicine* (9).

Chapter Five, on organic brain syndrome in the family, has been reprinted from a recent Symposium on Alzheimer's disease and related disorders, held at the University of California, Los Angeles. In this chapter an attempt is made to deal with "change" and "working through" on the level of the family system, in cases where the organic disorder usually remains unchanged. The family system, with its irrational role rigidities, displaced self-reproaches, paranoid fantasies, and fears of being overwhelmed, can be considered as a unit in relation to the health care system, which is not immune from reacting with similar irrational role rigidity, displaced self-reproaches, paranoid fantasies, and fears of being overwhelmed. The effective therapist must see therapeutic change on a supra-individual and supra-familial level that encompasses both family and health care systems. If this is not done, optimal work-up treatment and adjustment to illness may be severely compromised.

David Wellisch, drawing from vast experience with families of cancer patients, emphasizes many of the same issues in the final chapter. Wellisch dispels the notion that family treatment of the cancer patient, even the terminal one, is limited to dealing with death and dying. His rich case material illustrates poignantly the need for the therapist to facilitate the family's interactions with health care providers, the significance of marital dysfunction, the effects of parents' defenses on children, the special role of the terminal patient and obstacles posed by that specialness on communication within the family, and the dynamic issues behind the family search for unorthodox methods of treatment.

These chapters reflect only the beginnings of integrative treatment approaches that involve the family. The extent to which such approaches are necessary has, perhaps, been obscured by the classification of mental illness, which tends to imply that there actually exist isolable impairments of thinking, feeling (affective), conduct (personality), and body (somatic). In fact, most of these components must be considered in the treatment of most major disorders. The functions of thought, mood, conduct, and body are a great deal more dependent on interpersonal supports for their cohesion and intactness than is commonly acknowledged, even in the mental health field. There is a dearth of integrative thinking in most approaches to what are currently called personality disorders, whether or not they are accompanied by discrete symptoms, and affective disorders, whether psychotic or otherwise. Only integrative approaches that transcend reifications of disturbances of thinking, feeling, conduct, and body and place these disorders firmly in the context of close relationships (with defensive requirements of their own) can effectively cope with the multifaceted treatment requirements posed by major pathology.

Melvin R. Lansky, M.D.

References

1. Lansky MR (ed): Family Therapy and Major Psychopathology. New York, Grune & Stratton, 1981

2. Bateson G, Jackson D, Weakland J, et al: Toward a theory of schizophrenia. Behav Sci 1:251-264, 1956

3. Wynne L, Ryckoff I, Day J, et al: Pseudo-mutuality in the family relations of schizophrenics. Psychiatry 21:205-220, 1958

4. Bowen M: A family concept of schizophrenia, in The Etiology of Schizophrenia. Edited by Jackson D. New York, Basic Books, 1960

5. Lidz T, Fleck S, Cornelison A, et al: Schizophrenia and the Family. New York, International Universities Press, 1965

6. Bell N, Vogel E: The emotionally disturbed child as the family scapegoat, in The Psychosocial Interior of the Family. Edited by Handel G. Chicago, Aldine, 1967

7. Lansky MR: Family psychotherapy in the hospital, in Family Therapy and Major Psychopathology. Edited by Lansky MR. New York, Grune & Stratton, 1981

8. Kohut H: The Analysis of the Self. New York, International Universities Press, 1971

9. Block D: Family systems medicine: the field and the journal. Fam Systems Med 1:3-11, 1983

10. Lansky MR: The explanation of impulsive action. Int J Psychoanal Psychother (in press)

11. Brown G, Birley JLT, Wing JK: The influence of family life on the course of schizophrenic disorders: a replication. Br J Psychiatry 121:241-258, 1972

1

Masks of the Narcissistically Vulnerable Marriage

Melvin R. Lansky, M.D.

1

Masks of the Narcissistically Vulnerable Marriage

The Need for Disguise

Narcissistic vulnerability in marriage typically presents in a way that is disguised; even surface conflicts (say, over symptoms such as drinking, psychosis, or suicidality) are often screens deflecting attention from disorganizing propensities in the personalities of intact-seeming parties to the conflict. This need for disguise can usually be understood in terms of the narcissistic equilibrium of the group of people involved and their fear of exposure, fear of abandonment, and above all their vulnerability to humiliation. Shame dynamics are paramount in marriages manifesting narcissistic vulnerability, and the dread of being shamed is the main reason that marital difficulties have to be disguised. The awareness of narcissistic vulnerability is so mortifying that those with such vulnerability seek out intimate relationships or use those at hand in ways that will keep them from being exposed as fragmentation-prone or weak. A grossly symptomatic patient—for example, one with alcoholism, schizophrenia, or suicidality—may hide the vulnerabilities of an entire family. Disguise, however, is accom

---

Reprinted from International Journal of Family Psychiatry 3:439–419, 1983, with the kind permission of International Universities Press and Dr. John Howells, Editor-in-Chief.

plished only at the enormous cost of sustaining a very painful symptom or symptoms.

Treatment Failures

Treatment failure very commonly results from the therapist's neglecting to consider this narcissistic equilibrium within the family—that is, family members' needs to ward off exposure as inadequate, empty, or fragmentation-prone. I comment here on only a few among the many types of presentation that are prominent in my direct clinical experience.

Sex therapy. A retrospective study was made of treatment successes and failures in an unselected series of couples receiving conjoint treatment for sexual dysfunction (1). This study revealed that treatment failures were uniformly characterized by the presence of traits indicating narcissistic vulnerability in couples—that is, blaming, contempt, depression, and fears of intimacy. In the same sample the absence of these traits was uniformly associated with simple and uncomplicated symptom remission.

Depression. A sample of depressed hospitalized men, seen on admission to have endogenous or unipolar depressions with neurovegetative signs at the forefront, invariably improved on antidepressant medication to the point where neurovegetative signs and depressed mood improved (2, 3). A common finding in many of these patients was marriages typified by blaming transactions. Clinical depression was often compounded by blaming situations within the marriage, yet these conflictual marriages endured despite decades of unremitting misery. I comment on blaming marriages in a later section.

Impulsive symptomatic action. Close study of the familial relationships of those whose clinical picture is characterized by impulsive symptomatic action, such as self-poisoning, suicidality, wrist-slashing, alcoholism, and episodic violence, reveals that there is a typical precipitant (4). This is usually a disruption in an intimate relationship, which may set off a sequence of events in the individual that includes a fragmentation experience, often with a paranoid flavor and an urge to carry out an impulsive act. Such an act is often blamed by someone else in the family. The precipitating event may be, for example, a loss or rejection or a kind of emotional absence, withdrawal, or depression on the part of one spouse, which is immediately followed by, say, a drinking binge by the other. The drinking binge then serves as an invitation for blaming behavior by the first spouse. In that act of blaming there is an elevation in mood in the withdrawn spouse while he or she is actively blaming the other. Thus, the depression or fragmentation in one precipitates a kind of impulsive action in the alcoholic other, which then allows the first a chance to gain equilibrium by feeling angry, blaming, and self-righteous. This kind of relatedness—which underlies many impulsive actions, such as drinking, self-poisoning, slashing, promiscuity, and aggressiveness—can be best understood in terms of the narcissistic equilibrium in the relationship of the impulsive actor with a close family member.

Relapsing schizophrenia. It is a consistent research finding that a kind of narcissistic vulnerability in the behavior of family members of schizophrenics is associated with a worse-than-usual response to treatment and a high relapse rate. Characteristics designated as "negative affective style" (5) or high negative "expressed emotion" (6) include a kind of fusion of family members with the psychotic person and a mortifying type of blame, together with an inability of the family to separate from the patient with a psychosis and to lead lives of their own. Such traits are evidence of high narcissistic vulnerability. The family dynamics are similar in some ways to those of impulsive actors, and the psychotic behavior, like impulsive behavior, serves as a screen for narcissistic vulnerability in others in the family. This is not to say that the symptoms of schizophrenia are caused by the narcissistic needs of the family, but only that in some families psychotic propensities are provoked and exploited to regulate the narcissistic equilibrium of the family in a way that is associated with poor treatment response.

Drug discontinuance. The basis for drug discontinuance may go beyond the presence of side effects and include issues that can be understood in the context of the family and then overcome (7). For example, in some families taking medication may invite a view of the patient as defective, culpable, or blameworthy, and drug refusal may be understood as refusal to accept such a role. This is especially so if the physician is felt to be colluding with the family in blaming the patient for emotional turbulence. Or a schizophrenic whose sexual potency has been affected by the use of major tranquilizers may discontinue their use without discussing potency difficulties if he feels that his physician, like his family, believes that his sexuality is unimportant.

These situations have in common a symptomatic presentation that is at the forefront and a need for the maintenance of familial narcissistic equilibrium that is kept out of focus. The symptom is often the price—and a high one—for narcissistic equilibrium in family members, and such equilibrium is the major defensive concern of the whole family.

DEFENSIVE MANEUVERS

Symptoms often serve to justify defensive patterns that regulate distance in the family, that is, they keep family members from getting too close or too far away. Defensive patterns may give useful clues about the level of narcissistic pathology in the family. I comment on two types of familial defensive maneuvers that may not be recognized as such because they are hidden in the family's rationalizations. One type of defensive maneuver involving overt conflict but disguised cohesiveness is typified by blaming transactions and is indicative of severe pathology. Another type, which may be either mild or severe, is overtly cohesive, responsible, and caring but rationalizes chronic withdrawal as preoccupation with activities of great significance for the family. Both types involve collusion of the entire family.

Blame

Useful understanding of severe narcissistic vulnerability can be gained from considering typical transactions in chronically conflictual or blaming marriages. Blaming marriages may be distinguished from those that are not narcissistically vulnerable in a number of ways: In the blaming marriage, anger seems always present; one seemingly small issue after another—even if it is only a minor tardiness or defection of attention away from the other spouse—is used to justify the expression of infantile rage. In general, the spouses' unhappiness with the marriage is not resolvable even in principle, and the angry outbursts serve to let the spouses express the feelings that they are let down, injured, not cared for, and cheated. In marriages that are not characterized by severe narcissistic vulnerability, anger is usually confined to specific issues that the couples face; those issues may be taken at face value and are resolvable in principle. In blaming marriages there is an entitled, demanding, rageful insistence on justice that always goes beyond the issues being argued. In less vulnerable marriages the spouses can ask more directly and less self-righteously for what they want. In participants in blaming marriages one finds an early life history of intense trauma resulting either from frequent changes in nurturance or absence of emotional nurturance early in life; of involvement in an immature marriage as of the object of parentification, scapegoating, or blame; and often, of physical or sexual abuse with the knowledge of one or both parents. In marriages that are not severely vulnerable, disputes are usually based on different ideas of marriage (whether affirmed or rejected) that are derivatives of the parental marriages of each spouse. The partners feel that they can resolve the issues or that they can leave the marriage. Blaming couples feel empty, are absorbed in feeling injured and humiliated, and see real communication as a danger rather than an opportunity for improvement. With less vulnerable couples, ignorance, repression, and lack of communicative skills may play an important part in marital difficulties, and may be relieved by fairly simple means.

There is a vengeful, self-righteous quality about blaming couples, who usually regard the marriage as a shameful symbiosis and disown it completely—often to the point where they are unable to explain even to themselves why they are continually attached to a partner who is apparently so despicable. Less vulnerable couples, on the contrary, have a perspective on what is good about the relationship and a good deal of sadness that this may have to be sacrificed if what is bad cannot be resolved. Blaming marriages are characterized by a lack of observing ego, both partners being lost in the blaming transactions, almost as though these were different ego states. An observing ego is present in less vulnerable marriages. In blaming relationships, fusion shows up in the couple's use of discourse about "he," "she," or "we." There is more sense of separateness and the use of the word "I" in statements of spouses in less vulnerable marriages. Spouses in blaming marriages are invested not only in continued blaming but also in other symptomatology, such as drinking, suicidality, and dysfunction in children, and they draw others into the marriage. Marriages that are not characterized by vulnerability usually have enough of a sense of justice and personal cohesiveness to keep children from feeling responsible for the unhappiness. The latter point sheds light on a self-replicating quality of blaming marriages—namely, that they draw children into the conflict and predispose them to have the same pathology as the parents.

Preoccupation

A form of narcissistic vulnerability that can be more insidious is manifested by pathological preoccupation (8). Unlike blaming couples, who are usually in marriages characterized by irresponsibility, immaturity, and impulsive action and usually do not complain of specific marital difficulties, couples with pathologic preoccupation often appear close, caring, responsible, and, if anything, overwhelmed by their obligations, which they almost always keep. These obligations, however, justify and conceal an emotional absence, especially in intimate situations, that is rationalized by some other attachment, one with intense narcissistic value for the family: for example, attention to children (which may exert pressure on children to get this attention by being dysfunctional), the extended family, educational or professional advancement, community service, and so forth. The values justifying preoccupation may be shared so much that the preoccupation becomes system-syntonic. Couples with pathologic preoccupation do present with marital problems and often give the therapist the impression that they are fairly straightforward treatment cases. Despite early appearances, such cases often do not improve even after lengthy and skilled conjoint treatment. Often, one spouse does not complain about an extreme degree of preoccupation in the other; but even when the absence is justified, the preoccupation comes at a devastating price when the marriage is felt to be troubled, or a dysfunctional child may be in need of attention. The justified preoccupations are usually found to serve purposes of control and distance regulation and cannot be given up without making low-grade depressive traits much worse and flooding the preoccupied partners with humiliation. This type of narcissistic vulnerability with low-grade depressive features often becomes recognizable in the parental marriages of patients with attachment difficulties, impulsive action, or anorexia nervosa.

FEATURES OF NARCISSISTIC VULNERABILITY

Humiliation Proneness

Humiliation proneness is intense shame on being exposed as vulnerable, dependent, empty, and fragmentation-prone. This sense of shame is compounded by the feeling that those who point out what the family or the individuals in it are doing *intend* to shame them. In blaming marriages, responsibility for deficiencies that are shameful is felt by the blaming spouse to belong to the other. In the treatment situation, the therapist's attribution of any responsibility to the blaming spouse for the difficulties in the marriage may be experienced by that person as mortifying blame. This may be intolerable to the point that the person feeling blamed by the therapist may break off treatment. In marriages characterized by pathologic preoccupation, loyalties occupying the spouse's attention also offset their sense of shame. The spouse's feelings of worth in the family and out are buttressed by activities that raise their status or income or by being devoted parents. They are not founded on a cohesive feeling of self-worth that does not need such justification. Exploration of these issues may be followed by missed sessions justified by other responsibilities. Humiliation proneness is a major source of unconscious resistance by patients in any type of treatment and a deterrent to any simple solution of symptom removal in the narcissistically vulnerable. Indeed, the types of treatment failure noted earlier were all situations in which brief sexual therapy, antidepressants, Antabuse, phenothiazines, simple counseling, psychotherapy, or marital therapy had been tried and had failed to accomplish full symptomatic remission.

Evidence of Pathologic Distance Regulation

This refers to relationships organized around avoiding separateness on the part of the members but at the same time avoiding intimacy (8). Such distance regulation deals both with the dread of separation and that of being exposed as weak or inadequate. In blaming marriages, intimacy is avoided by a hostile verbal attack that avoids closeness but also keeps the couple's attention exclusively on the relationship. In preoccupied states, a close-knit marital situation is offset by inattention and emotional withdrawal rationalized as divided loyalty.

Fusion

Fusion is a reliable indication of pathologic distance regulation. Fusion involves the use of collusive transpersonal defenses—for example, pathologic projective identification that imputes to and provokes in others traits which are participated in vicariously but also disowned (9). In blaming transactions, lack of separateness is explicit in the reproach that the blamer has been betrayed, cheated, abandoned, or let down and implicit in the provocations and invitations to engage in blameworthy behavior. In preoccupied states, activities separate from the marriage must be justified as being necessitated by another loyalty that is important to the marriage (e.g., children, educational, or vocational advancement). Spouses in pathologically preoccupied marriages seldom seek separate gratifications that are not justified as duties.

TREATMENT

There is a good deal of reluctance on the part of family therapists to acknowledge that narcissistic personality organization poses special problems in the treatment of families and to face the complex treatment problems involved with such pathology. If the therapist is only comfortable conceptualizing and administering treatment for presenting symptomatology, that therapist may collude with the family in avoiding scrutiny of narcissistic vulnerability. Nonetheless, in many kinds of symptom presentations—ranging from marital misery to dysfunction in a child, impulsive action, or depression—severe narcissistic vulnerability has to be contended with to avoid treatment failure. The treatment of narcissistic vulnerability in marriages is incompletely developed, and only a few treatment strategies can be set forward at this time. Below are listed some major obstacles opposing change and indicated treatment approaches for contending with them:

1. *Transpersonal defensive operations.* The symptomatic presentation often is so system-syntonic or the narcissistic mission of the family is so in accord with common defensive concerns that defensive operations go beyond one person, and the whole family participates. When the transpersonal defenses show up in excess reactivity (e.g., blaming) rather than inhibition, one must use a style of family therapy that does not encourage people to react to one another, but rather the reverse—to pull back from reactivity. This may be accomplished by having all transactions go through the therapist, as Bowen has advocated (10).
2. *Humiliation proneness.* This trait is at the center of narcissistic vulnerability. Often the therapist can reduce it by interfering

with reactivity that is based on feelings of inadequacy. The use of intergenerational reconstructions that point to the unfolding history of the preoccupations—for example, fear of being left or being out of control or being helpless—may be a specific technique for the handling of intense shame on being exposed as one who is afraid of abandonment or needs to control or avoids helplessness.

3. *The need for distance regulation*. Controlling maneuvers of the patient often become the occasion for intense resentment by therapists or countermaneuvers to get around them (11). With narcissistic vulnerability, some sort of distance regulation—some sort of control over people so that they are not too close and not too far away—is a necessity. It is to the advantage of the treatment to acknowledge this defensive need, to point to the struggle, and to open the whole issue up for discussion rather than to blame the system and the patients for needing to regulate distance. The therapist's need to countercontrol is an obvious impediment to treatment.
4. *Emotional holding*. Patients with narcissistic vulnerability need a low-risk empathic situation where the fear of getting too close or getting too far away is minimal. This may not necessarily be in the same setting as the treatment situation in which conflicts are explored with the spouse. Psychoanalysis (for the few for whom it is feasible) may provide both opportunities. Multiple-family group therapy (2) is a neglected mode of therapy but may also supply both conflict resolution and emotional constancy. Conjoint family therapy alone is not necessarily the treatment of choice for narcissistically vulnerable persons in a marriage (12). Need for distance regulation, use of collusive defenses, and humiliation proneness require combinations and treatment strategies that are administered mindful of these difficulties and devised to deal with the specific pathological predicaments rather than a simplification suited to the preferences of the therapist.

References

1. Lansky MR, Davenport AE: Difficulties in brief conjoint treatment of sexual dysfunction. Am J Psychiatry 132:177–179, 1975

2. Lansky MR, Bley CR, McVey G: Multiple family groups as after care. Int J Group Psychother 28:211–224, 1978

3. Lansky MR: On Blame. Int J Psychoanal Psychother 8:429–456, 1980

4. Lansky MR: The explanation of impulsive action. Int J Psychoanal Psychother (in press)

5. West KL: The assessment and treatment of disturbed adolescents and their families: a clinical research perspective, in Family Therapy and Major Psychopathology. Edited by Lansky MR. New York, Grune & Stratton, 1981

6. Brown GW, Birley JLT, Wing JK: The influence of family life on the course of schizophrenia: a replication. Br J Psychiatry 121:241–258, 1972

7. Lansky MR: Medication and family process, in Family Therapy and Major Psychopathology. Edited by Lansky MR. New York, Grune & Stratton, 1981

8. Lansky MR: Preoccupation and pathologic distance regulation. Int J Psychoanal Psychother, vol. 11, 1985

9. Johnson A, Szurek S: The genesis of antisocial acting out in children and adults. Psychoanal Q 21:323–343, 1952

10. Bowen M: The use of family theory in clinical practice. Compr Psychiatry 7:345–379, 1966

11. Lansky MR: The role of the family in the evaluation of suicidality. Int J Fam Psychiatry 3:105–118, 1982

12. Lansky MR: Treatment of the narcissistically vulnerable marriage, in Family Therapy and Major Psychopathology. Edited by Lansky MR. New York, Grune & Stratton, 1981

2

Families and Family Therapy in Alcoholism

Edward Kaufman, M.D.

2

Families and Family Therapy in Alcoholism

Family therapists and family system researchers have recently contributed substantially to the rapidly growing knowledge and expertise in the field of alcoholism. Although the family of the alcoholic has received a great deal of attention over the past 30 years, only recently have quantitative, objective, comparative studies of role relationships and interaction patterns in families with an alcoholic member been presented. These recent studies, which will be summarized here, demonstrate the following aspects of these families:

1. a high incidence of familial alcoholism, depression, and disruption;
2. depression and stress-related medical illness in spouses;
3. a high incidence of blaming, competition for dominance, and responsibility avoidance in alcoholics;
4. a high incidence of negative affect in alcoholic-spouse interactions.

The recent concern given to factors other than alcoholism which influence these family systems—including social class, ethnicity, gender of the identified patient, psychopathology in other members, and changes based on the family life cycle and phases of reactivity—will also be discussed. Finally, some workable programs that have been developed for the therapy of alcoholic families will be presented.

QUANTITATIVE STUDIES OF ALCOHOLISM AND THE FAMILY

Familial Alcoholism and Depression

The high incidence of familial alcoholism and depression in alcoholics is one of the oldest and most frequently replicated findings in these families. Cotton's (1) review of 39 studies in the literature found that 27 percent of the fathers of alcoholics and five percent of the mothers were themselves alcoholic.

The families of female alcoholics are generally found to have more alcoholism and depression than those of males. In a study by Lisansky (2), 44 percent of alcoholic women and 35 percent of alcoholic men gave a history of a parent with excessive drinking. Sherfey (3) found that 68 percent of women with alcoholism came from homes with alcoholism as opposed to 45 percent of men, and Bromet and Moos's study (4) similarly reported that female alcoholics have more heavy-drinking mothers than male alcoholics.

Winokur and Clayton's (5) study of the families of 69 male and 45 female alcoholics revealed that women alcoholics have a higher prevalence of alcoholism in their fathers (28 percent), mothers (12 percent), and female siblings (12 percent) than male alcoholics (21 percent, three percent, two percent respectively). They also found that affective illness was more common in the fathers (six percent) of female alcoholics than in their mothers (two percent), although other types of psychiatric illnesses were more common in mothers. Later studies of younger female alcoholics show a substantial increase in maternal alcoholism with lowered age of the alcoholic, which may be indicative of recent future increases in alcoholism in women (6).

In her literature review, Beckman (7) noted that despite one unusually low estimate of six percent, estimates of prevalence of alcoholism in the fathers of women alcoholics ranged from 28 percent to 50 percent.

It is generally accepted that a substantial part of the relationship between parental alcoholism and depression and alcoholism in progeny is a result of genetic transmission. Danish studies by Goodwin et al. (8) showed that progeny adopted away from alcoholics were four times more likely than controls to develop alcoholism. Nevertheless, there is also general agreement that nongenetic factors, such as sociocultural influences, role modeling, and childhood stress levels from growing up in an alcoholic home, also contribute to alcoholism (9–11). Wolin et al. (12) have noted that the description of key family rituals from one generation to the next is associated with greater intergenerational recurrence of alcoholism.

Winokur et al. (13), in a study of families of alcoholics, found a 15.5 percent chance of depression and a 15.1 percent chance of alcoholism in first-degree relatives. The same group (14) also noticed a tendency for male alcoholics to have female relatives with a depressive disorder. Since it is so common, Winokur termed depression associated with first-degree family history of alcoholism, "depressive-spectrum disease"; in his study it was more common in women.

Another common finding in the families of female alcoholics is an emotionally brutal childhood with a high incidence of familial disruption. In a study by Sandmaier (15), problem-drinking women were more likely than men to have lost one of their parents through divorce, desertion, or death during their childhood. Wilsnack (16), too, noted that alcoholic women have a high rate of family disruption, including loss of one or both parents through death, divorce, or separation, and alcoholism or psychosis in parents or close relatives. Gomberg (17) reported that although the rates of such disruption are high in both alcoholic men and women, they are higher in women. Women who have experienced broken homes before the age of 10 are significantly more likely than men with the same history to become heavy drinkers (18).

Depression and Stress-Related Illnesses in Spouses

In a study of alcoholics and their spouses as compared to a matched control group, Moos et al. (19) found the following characteristics of spouses of alcoholics: more alcohol consumption, more negative life events, fewer social and recreational activities, less family cohesiveness, more depression, more medical conditions, and more job changes. Moos et al. also noted that when the alcoholic controlled drinking, the negative effects on the spouse diminished. The findings by Moos are in marked contrast to the earlier literature in the field of alcoholism and the family, which emphasized the wife's need to keep the alcoholic sick and her decompensation when the alcoholic became sober (11). Moos's quantitative study also confirms the conclusion reached by Edwards et al. (20) after their extensive review of the literature—that dysfunction in the wives of alcoholics tends to disappear when the stresses of living with a drinking alcoholic are dissipated. Similarly, Orford et al. (21) found that after one year of drastic reduction in drinking, there was an increase in husband-to-wife affection and a nonsignificant increase in wife-to-husband affection. Interestingly, Orford's good outcome group was characterized by five times as many husband-dominated or egalitarian couples than the bad outcome group.

On the other hand, Jacob et al. (22) reported that the female spouses of male alcoholics who drank steadily had higher satisfaction and reduced symptoms associated with higher alcohol consumption in their mates. However, this was not true of female spouses of binge alcoholics, a finding that may be related to the binge drinkers' much higher incidence of fighting, job loss, family neglect, and arrests for drunken behavior. Jacob's work emphasizes the need for looking at subtypes of alcoholic families before making generalizations. Steinglass's (23) studies of the adaptive consequences of drinking are consistent with the homeostatic need of some families of alcoholics to perpetuate alcoholism, and also emphasize the need to examine different types and stages of alcoholic families.

Blaming, Competition for Dominance, and Responsibility Avoidance

Gorad (24) has shown that male alcoholics exceed their wives, normal husbands, and normal wives in the use of responsibility-avoiding messages. Further, both the alcoholic and his wife are highly competitive in style, using more "one-up" messages and cooperating less than other couples.

Orford et al. (25) found that in alcoholic families, particularly those with a poor prognosis, the wives gave and received little affection; wives used few socially desirable adjectives in describing their "sober" husband; and wives expected their husbands to use "hostile-dominance" adjectives or phrases.

Chiles et al. (26) compared alcoholic couples with sexual dysfunction with a control group of non-alcoholic couples with sexual dysfunction. Although they did not find significant differences in wives' dominance as described by either husbands or wives, alcoholic husbands saw themselves as submissive (the wives disagreed). They suggest that male alcoholics feel submissive because of their own needs to misperceive the situation, not because their wives are dominant and force them into submission. My own clinical experience with these families is that both husbands and wives consistently feel dominated by each other.

Gorad (24) has commented that the alcoholic's wife appears dominating because she is responsible and direct. However, she is unable to control her husband, and unfortunately for treatment, neither spouse accepts that the other will ever change. Paolino and McCrady (27) have noted that these couples will blame each other, put each other down, turn each other off, and compete for dominance. They sidetrack each other and then terminate communication without a solution, leading to the alcoholic's fleeing the scene to drink.

Billings et al. (28) found that the marital interactions of alcoholics and their wives were more pathologic than those of nondistressed couples but did not differ significantly from those of non-alcoholic but distressed couples. Specifically, both alcoholic and distressed couples had more negative and hostile acts and fewer rational problem-solving statements.

Negative Affect in Spousal Relations

Jacob et al. (29) studied alcoholic families compared to normals, both sober and under the influence of alcohol. In this study, alcoholic-spouse interactions had more negative affect, which increased in the presence of alcohol, and alcoholic fathers showed less leadership, assertiveness, and problem-solving behavior with spouse and children.

Many other aspects of the family of the alcoholic have been described but not yet quantitatively documented (11). Although the studies I have described in this section are all based on quantitative measures and many have used matched control groups, there is an almost absolute lack of comparison between families with an alcoholic member and other types of dysfunctional families. The exceptions are the work of Chiles et al. (26) and Billings et al. (28), which may be particularly similar to those of alcoholics. Thus, families worthy of comparative study would include those with a parent with a borderline personality disorder, prescription drug abuse, depression particularly with frequent suicide attempts, severe jealousy, and constant repetitive quarreling.

FACTORS OTHER THAN ALCOHOLISM WHICH INFLUENCE THE ALCOHOLIC FAMILY SYSTEMS

Social Class and Ethnicity

A family's social class and ethnic influences may play a bigger role in the family's adaptive and maladaptive patterns than the symptoms (alcoholism and related behavior) of the identified patient—or, to use a family systems term, Index Patient (IP). Social class and ethnicity may also govern family attitudes toward drinking behavior that may contribute to alcohol use, abuse, and alcoholism.

It is also necessary to take into consideration many different variables within each ethnic group. Nevertheless, there are ethnic patterns in alcoholic families which illustrate the overall significance of ethnic family style in alcoholism problems. The following portraits are intended to highlight commonly observed ethnic features that should be considered in overall treatment approaches and are commonly neglected. They are deliberately oversimplified and are not meant to be stereotypes that apply to all members of the ethnic groups under consideration.

Irish-American alcoholic family patterns are substantially influenced by ethnic factors. Irish-American families are skillful with words but are usually not in touch with their feelings (30). The Irish often drink for reassurance and to escape from burdens of guilt and the need to repress sexuality and aggression. Irish families are frequently ruled by domineering, matriarchal mothers, who continue their dominance of the family even when the children are middle-aged. Thus, one would expect Irish mothers to exert strong influences over their sons and grandsons, and a general lack of separation of all family members from their family of origin (31). This can produce marital strains, which are worsened by cultural encouragement of procreation and strictures against birth control that lead to the production of children before couples work out their dyadic relationship (32).

Many Irish fathers in inner cities work extra jobs and evening hours in positions such as policemen, which means that they spend little time with the family. In addition, these fathers have a strong, role-oriented peer group that influences their functions and values and supports their alcoholism. A family structure with such an absentee father accentuates the tendency for the mother to be responsible for and over-involved with family functions and tasks.

In Italian-American families, too, there are intense ties from all family members, particularly males, to their family of origin, which prevent them from relating closely and without constant interference to their families of procreation (33). The white Anglo-Saxon family tends to place a strong emphasis on independence, which can at times extrude children from the family early and weaken the ties to the extended family. They sometimes have difficulties in communication and are emotionally bland, with an inadequate sense of self-worth, particularly when they do not meet the expectations of the Calvinistic work ethic (34). In Jewish families one observed pattern includes an attempt at consensual democracy, with the entire family enmeshed and substantial guilt provocation—the price for autonomy and independence (33).

The constant impact of racism and discrimination is a continuing and pervasive aspect of the black family system. Thus, alcoholism is rampant in black ghetto families, with a rate of 48 percent in black males and a high ratio of female alcoholism as well (35).

Although females lead more black families than white families, the two-parent family is still the norm among American blacks. However, there is more role flexibility among black two-parent families, with black fathers playing a larger role in child rearing and nurturing than white fathers (32).

Discipline of children is strict and direct, but the lack of positive support by social structures leads to a high incidence of substance abuse in youth.

The specific variations in the treatment techniques that are used with these different ethnic groups are discussed under the family therapy section.

Gender of the Identified Patient

Until recently, alcoholics have been written about as if they were all males, with relatively little attention paid to the specific nature of the personality, psychopathology, and family aspects of the female.

In certain specific ways, families of female alcoholics are consistently quite different from families of male alcoholics. Of course, individual differences are critical and modify the influence of such generalizations.

Women tend to hide their drinking from their families, and the families in turn tend to deny drinking by their maternal figure (7). Drinking by women is very much related to the problems of nonalcoholic women in our society, such as lack of social power and the external pressure they experience to suppress aspects of selves which do not conform to female sex stereotypes (15).

However, when female alcoholics compare themselves to non-alcoholic women, the alcoholics see themselves as less socially competent and less effective in goal achievement. They have more covert and overt anxiety and feel unworthy and dissatisfied with their purpose in life (36). They also have more depression than male alcoholics, as discussed previously (5, 37).

Family of origin in female alcoholics. Many women alcoholics perceive that they had cold, severe, bossy, domineering mothers and warmer, gentle, but alcoholic fathers (7). These fathers only rebel against their dominant wives when they are drunk. The pre-alcoholic daughters tend to reject their parents, particularly their mothers. Daughters in such families feel that the alcoholic father prefers them to the mother, and that if mother were more loving, father would not drink. They gravitate to their fathers for the affection and support they feel they do not receive from their mothers. Because they also identify with their alcoholic fathers, they are directly vulnerable to developing alcoholism as adults and to marrying alcoholics, even in repeated marriages (38).

Although the pattern of a weak father who is over-involved with his pre-alcoholic daughter is common, the totally absent father is also rather prevalent.

Nuclear family. Female alcoholics have a high divorce rate, as their husbands leave them more frequently than wives leave male alcoholics (6); the economic dependence of wives on husbands undoubtedly plays a role here. They are also more likely to be married to a fellow alcoholic (7).

The husbands of female alcoholics may initially deny that their wives drink, perhaps because these women hide it so well or are so neglected that the husband does not notice the drinking. In some families, husbands may be quite critical and rejecting of wives' drinking. Later, they may abandon their wives, or continue to live with them as "co-alcoholics" whose own lives are totally preoccupied with the spouse and her drinking. Co-alcoholics unconsciously collude to perpetuate the alcoholism.

Generally, men are much less nurturing than women and are less willing to nurse along a sick alcoholic spouse. Husbands who continue to live with alcoholic wives may also have extremely high levels of denial, so that they experience neither frustration nor depression (39).

Alcoholic women also have sexual problems, including orgastic dysfunction (40), but not the general promiscuity that was reported in the early literature.

If both spouses misuse alcohol, they tend to form a supportive network which assists each of them in continuing on the path of alcoholism. Despite this overt support, these relationships are rarely loving and eventually deteriorate (38).

Role as mother. Not all female alcoholics are grossly inadequate mothers, as the mothering function is the last aspect of social functioning that is lost. However, 57 percent of the married women in Corrigan's study (6) had difficulty in their role as wife, and 42 percent had difficulty in their role as mother, with 44 percent and 32 percent respectively stating they were unable to fulfill these roles at all. In the same study, 80 percent of the alcoholic women raised their own children, but 39 percent had been separated from their children for prolonged periods.

Whereas alcoholic fathers tend to abuse their children sexually and violently, alcoholic mothers are more prone to abuse their children through neglect. Thus children of alcoholic mothers tend to be cold, distrustful, rigid, and reserved, submissive, and dependent, like their mothers (41), and to have learning difficulties and school problems (6).

Therapists should, of course, not react to women in terms of cultural stereotypes but should be sensitive to the specific problems of women substance abusers in our society and address these issues in treatment. These issues will be addressed under the family psychotherapy section of this chapter.

Stage of Alcoholism and the Family

With the exceptions of Steinglass (23), Jackson (42), and Kaufman and Pattison (11), most studies of the families of alcoholics have not addressed the issue of the differential effects of various phases of substance use on the family system. After an initial phase of denial, but still early in an Index Patient's (IP's) alcohol abuse, families tend to overreact in an enmeshed and chaotic way to alcohol-related behavior, particularly during intoxication and heavy use. Later on, there is usually more of a tendency to exclude the IP and form a new homeostasis without him or her. Unfortunately, some families may stay enmeshed and fused to the IP, and family members may be dragged down to severe depression and substance abuse themselves. Families may also cycle from disengagement to enmeshed reactivity and then back to emotionally and physically separated stages. There are even some families who are relatively unaffected by alcoholism, either because the alcoholism is walled off outside of the family system or because of a working homeostasis which protects the alcoholic and family. These families are resistant to intensive or restructuring family therapy (11).

A Workable System of Family Therapy for Alcoholics

Every therapist's system of family therapy should be a Personal Evolving Method of Therapy (PEMT) (43). A workable system of family therapy includes basic rules of thumb and specific adaptations of family therapy techniques to meet the needs of alcoholics and their families.

Basic Rules of Thumb of Treatment

1. Simple, direct courses of action are most helpful.
2. A basic knowledge of the medical, social, and psychological aspects of alcoholism and associated common family systems is essential.

3. An assessment of the extent of alcohol use and alcoholism is necessary in order to determine the therapeutic stance in relation to alcohol.
4. A system of developing a substance-free state must be established early.
5. A system must be established for maintaining an alcohol-free state.
6. Working with the family must continue where substance abuse continues.

It is important in the first session or two that the therapist evaluate the extent of the alcoholism and the difficulties it presents for the individual and family. This history is generally taken with the entire family present, as alcoholics will often be honest in this setting, and their "confession" is a helpful way to begin communication. On the other hand, other family members can often provide more accurate information than the IP, and some IPs will give an accurate history only when interviewed alone. In taking an alcoholism history it is important to know what use has been made of every type of abusable drug as well as alcohol, including quantity, quality, duration, expense, how intake was supported and prevented, physical effects, tolerance, withdrawal, and medical complications. Only when the use of alcohol and other drugs has been quantified can the specific system necessary to achieve abstinence be decided upon (38).

As basic rule 4 indicates, it is critically important to establish a system early that enables the alcoholic or alcohol abuser to become sober to a point where family therapy can take place effectively. The specific methods employed to achieve this vary on a continuum according to the extent of use, abuse, and dependence. Often, mild to moderate alcohol abuse in adolescents can be controlled if both parents can agree on clear limits and expectations and how to enforce them. Older alcohol abusers may also stop using if they are made aware of the medical or psychological consequences to themselves or the effects on their family system (38).

If abuse has progressed, more aggressive methods are necessary to establish an alcohol-free system. If the alcoholic's intake is so severe that he or she is unable to attend sessions without being under the influence, if social or vocational functioning is severely impaired, if there is alcohol-related violence, or if there is physical dependence, the first priority in treatment is to stop substance abuse immediately. Then the goal is to persuade the family to pull together to initiate detoxification or at least some measure to achieve temporary abstinence. Generally, this is best done in a hospital; if the abuse pattern is severe, hospitalization will be required in the first session or very early in the therapy.

Once free of alcohol abuse, the family is urged to adopt some system which will enable them to continue to stay free of alcohol and other abuse substances, and this system is part of the therapeutic contract made early in treatment. A lifetime commitment to abstinence is not required, but the "one day at a time" approach of Alcoholics Anonymous (AA) is recommended, in which the alcoholic is asked to establish a system for abstinence which he or she commits to for only one day at a time but which he or she is reminded of daily by the basic principle of AA.

If the IP is or has ever been physically dependent, the family is informed that therapy is generally quite successful when they work toward abstinence and almost never works if controlled drinking is their goal. One specific problem with the approach of controlled drinking or substance use is that the individual cannot take advantage of AA as a support group while continuing to use abusable substances. Many people new to AA will have to shop for AA groups in which they feel personally comfortable. Every recovering alcoholic is strongly encouraged to attend small study groups that work on the well known twelve steps of AA, as well as their larger speaker meetings.

Many alcoholics will require hospitalization in a specialized alcohol treatment unit to reinforce their awareness of their need for AA and to provide a 24-hour-a-day intensive educational, supportive, and confrontational approach to their alcoholism and its physical and social consequences.

Some families will not accept hospitalization of the alcoholic until other methods have failed. In order to persuade them of the need for hospitalization, a therapist may have to maintain long-term ties with the family, even through multiple treatment failures. On the other hand, it may be more helpful to terminate treatment if the alcoholic continues to drink, rather than continue treatment which offers the family the pretense of change in a situation where no improvement is occurring. This excludes temporary "slips" into alcohol use, which are an expected part of the treatment. Treatment should not be terminated as a result of a few "slips" but should be ended if the family does not adopt any workable system for enforcing abstinence. When the therapist has properly joined with such families and they truly believe that treatment is being terminated in their best interest, they invariably return to treatment a few months or years later, ready and willing to commit to abstinence.

In some families in which alcohol abuse continues, despite the best efforts of the family therapist, a system of family therapy continues to be necessary whether or not the alcoholic enters into or remains in treatment. The first method to be considered in such circumstances is an intervention developed by Vernon Johnson (44). The therapist meets with everyone in the immediate family and significant members of the alcoholic's network, particularly employees and peers. The family is coached, through role playing, to confront the alcoholic with his or her behavior with concern and factual information and without hostility. The family and network are also advised to present firmly the consequences of continued alcoholism (job loss, divorce, etc.) and to have a viable alternative (AA, hospitalization with knowledge of insurance, etc.).

If this intervention is not used or is unsuccessful, then the therapist is faced with the common problem of working with the family without the alcoholic present. Here the family is strongly encouraged to attend Al-Anon, Alateen, and significant other groups to provide the support necessary to live with an alcoholic, particularly without being drawn back into cycles of alcohol-perpetuating behavior and personal despair (co-alcoholism). Family members are also given three choices: 1) Continue to do what you are doing, 2) emotionally detach, 3) move out or have the alcoholic move out (45). Therapy then is involved with diminishing the family's feelings of helplessness and helping them to make active choices.

Family Therapy Techniques

The family therapy techniques used with alcoholic families are a synthesis of structural and psychodynamic family therapy (11, 38). These have been described in detail elsewhere and will be discussed here only in the context of modification to meet the needs of alcoholic families. The techniques discussed include the contract, joining, actualization, marking boundaries, tasks, reframing, paradox, balancing and unbalancing, and psychodynamic approaches.

The therapeutic contract. The contract, which is made at the end of the first or second session, should focus on alcohol use and abuse and how the family should deal with and react to it. It should specify the system which the IP will use to detoxify and to maintain abstinence. In addition, the family's involvement in support groups such as Alanon or a multifamily group should also be made a part of the contract, and the family members should be provided with a method to deal with their emotionality about alcohol-related behaviors. As part of the contract, they may be coached either to disengage from their reactivity to substance use or, paradoxically, to monitor it more closely.

Joining. In joining (46), the therapist 1) reinforces areas of family strength, 2) rewards and affiliates with each family member, 3) complements and supports threatened members, and 4) explains problems. In doing so, the therapist uses the family's metaphors, expressions, and language. He or she alternates between joining that supports the family system and its members and different techniques that challenge them. The therapist must be alert to the possibility that joining with one part of a family system may severely stress or change the rest of that system.

In joining with the family, the therapist must alternate between existential engagement and disengaged expertness, and must be capable of joining each subsystem, including the siblings. The family members should feel the therapist's respect for each of them as individuals, as well as his firm commitment to healing. The therapist enters the family as a supporter of family rules but makes the rules work in the direction of therapeutic goals (38).

A knowledge of AA and Al-Anon is essential when working with families who have experience with these helpful organizations. AlAnon members have learned to "release with love" and can use this metaphor to help them disengage from an alcohol-abusing child or spouse.

Ultimately, the most significant joining occurs when the therapist communicates to the family that he or she understands them and is working with and for them. Thus, paradoxically, the most profound joining comes when the therapist challenges the family's dysfunctional maneuvers, which gives them hope that the therapist can make them better.

It is often difficult to join every member of the family, particularly drinking alcoholics, who can best be joined by a recovering alcoholic.

Actualizing family transactional patterns. Patients usually direct their communications to the therapist (47). They should be trained to talk to each other rather than to the therapist, and to enact transactional patterns rather than describe them.

When a therapist finds himself bored with a session, it is frequently because actualization (or change) has not occurred. Alcoholic families frequently gravitate to a rehash of past fights, hoping to entrap the therapist into deciding who started the fight, who is wrong and right, and what the proper resolution is. It is critical not to be triangulated into such a position, but rather to have the family choose an as yet unresolved conflict and actualize its problem-solving methods or lack of them in the session. If a family arrives with an intoxicated member they should not be dismissed, but their interactions should be observed; this will demonstrate how they interact during a good proportion of their time together.

Of course, if intoxication is a repeated problem, then the family must renegotiate a system to end the substance abuse.

Marking boundaries. One critical boundary which must be maintained or restored is that which protects the spousal system from interference from children, in-laws, or lovers (47). This may not be possible until alcohol intake is controlled. A helpful principle, which may even be a part of the therapeutic contract, is the rule of preservation of individual boundaries—for example, no one talks, feels, thinks, answers, or acts for another. Further, individuals are encouraged to tell their own story, own their own memory, and not interrupt each other. Individuals should be talked to and not about, and should listen to and acknowledge the communications of others. Nonverbal checking and blocking of communications should also be observed and, when appropriate, pointed out and halted. "Mind reading" is very common in these families and is strongly discouraged; even if the mind reader is correct, such behavior almost always starts an argument because no one likes to be anticipated in his reactions. Although not essential, Al-Anon and Alateen may be helpful in reinforcing the necessary disengagement of family members who are enmeshed with the alcoholic.

Assigning tasks. Tasks are perhaps the most important technique in family therapy, representing the major road to change in much the same way that transference does in individual psychoanalytic psychotherapy. Tasks intensify the relationship with the therapist and continue the therapeutic change process outside of the session (48).

Initial tasks should mesh with the family's goals, particularly those which correct the presenting symptoms of the IP. Tasks should be quite specific and should be given clearly, concisely, and firmly at the end of each session. They should be reviewed at the beginning of the following session and used as learning experiences if they failed. If performed successfully, they are building blocks for further change.

Reframing. Reframing is frequently used to shift behavior to a more positive light or normalize it (47). Thus, adolescent rebelliousness that produces parental overreaction can be labeled as normal individuation. A couple's constant battling can be interpreted as a result of the intense need both have for each other's love. Behavior may be reframed in order to broaden its focus—from the IP to the family, from problems at work to problems in the home, from alcoholism to intrafamilial problems. Problems and failures can be reframed as learning experiences.

The paradox. Paradoxical techniques are commonly used with alcoholic families, perhaps to the point where they have been over-utilized. In paradox the therapist gives an overt instruction in such a manner that the IP or family does the opposite, thus enabling the therapist to achieve his covert aim. One explanation for their popularity is that paradoxical techniques work best with chronic, rigid, repetitive, circular, highly resistant family systems, particularly those that have had many prior therapeutic failures (49).

One should not prescribe an individual's behavior without relating it to its function in the family system. A symptom should only be prescribed if its functions in the system are understood and it is prescribed in a way which changes the functioning of the system (49). This type of technique is a way of making a psychodynamic or systems interpretation that paradoxically gives the family added impetus to change behavior.

Balancing and unbalancing. Balancing techniques tend to support a family and unbalancing to stress the family system. As a family changes, the therapist moves between balancing and unbalancing. Balancing is similar to Minuchin and Fishman's complementarity (50). Thus, balancing challenges the family's views of symptoms as part of a linear hierarchy and emphasizes the reciprocal involvement in symptom formation.

When the therapist interprets behavior in this context, mutual responsibility is emphasized and tasks are given which involve change in both parties. The therapist must be aware that some individuals' views of their contributions are so skewed that what the therapist believes is well balanced may seem very unbalanced and unfair to them.

Unbalancing involves changing the existing hierarchy in a family and should be done only after the therapist has a great deal of power through joining. The therapist unbalances by affiliating with family members of lower power so that the latter can challenge their prescribed family role (50). The therapist may also paradoxically unbalance by affiliating with a dominant member in order to elicit a challenging response from those of less power. The therapist's affiliation in the family unbalances and interrupts rigid, repetitive cycles.

Psychodynamic concepts and techniques. Psychodynamic techniques use the past to change the present and focus on unconscious thought processes in every family member and the therapist. The symptom of the IP is viewed in the context of his or her own historical past and that of every family member. Psychodynamic family therapy has an ultimate goal in common with strategic therapies—that of achieving second-order change. Thus, the goal is to change the entire family system so that dysfunction does not occur in other family members when the symptoms of the IP are alleviated.

Psychodynamic techniques can be particularly useful when they are applied to the present in a here-and-now way. The past is explored only to change the future. The past is not dwelled on to rationalize behavior or to replay old patterns of guilt induction and hostility. Some families live their present in past events and feelings. They can deal with the present only after they have expunged their past hurts.

There are two cornerstones for the implementation of psychodynamic techniques: the therapist's knowledge of self and a detailed family history. The concepts basic to the effective use of psychodynamic techniques—countertransference, interpretation, resistance, and working through—will be discussed in terms of their use in family therapy.

Countertransference plays a special role in family therapy, as is often clear during supervision when the therapist is unable to utilize the supervisor's suggestions. A therapist may have countertransference reactions about many aspects of a patient and his or her family other than their transferences to the therapist.

Therapists may have specific types of emotional reactions to alcoholics and their families. The IP's dependency, relationship suctions and repulsions, manipulativeness, denial, impulsivity, and role abandonment will provoke countertransference reactions in the therapist depending on his or her own emotional makeup. However, family therapists must view their emotional reactions to families in a systems framework as well as a countertransference context. Thus, they must be aware of how these families will replay their problems with the therapist by attempting to detour or triangulate their problems to him. In these families, the therapist must be particularly sensitive about becoming a co-alcoholic, who tries to protect or is provoked to reject the alcoholic. One example of replication in the relationship between the therapist and the family of what happens within the family at home occurs when the therapist alternates between saving and persecution, first allowing the alcoholic to do almost anything, even coming drunk to sessions, and then switching to a punitive position, such as demanding sobriety before allowing the alcoholic to come to therapy. In addition to recognizing the meaning of such situations, the therapist must distinguish countertransference from a more generalized negativism or hostility toward substance abusers. Both are antitherapeutic (38).

Interpretations can be extremely helpful if they are used without blaming, guilt induction, or dwelling on the hopelessness of long-standing, fixed patterns. The repetitive patterns and their derivatives, and their maladaptive aspects, are pointed out to the patient and family, and they are given tasks to help them change these patterns in the here and now. Some families need interpretations before they can fulfill tasks. These are usually made in a complementary way, identifying each member's role in the family behaviors. An emphasis on complementary responsibility when making an interpretation is an example of the helpful fusion of structural and psychodynamic therapy (38).

In families with an alcoholic member, key resistance behaviors which must be dealt with involve the failure to perform system functions related to maintaining abstinence. Some resistances are often fixed in these patients—for example, parent-IP coalitions and triangulated parental conflict. Thus it is important to understand these resistances and to have methods for overcoming them.

When work with these families begins, the initial treatment contract can focus on the family's resistance, specifying that each family member agrees to cooperate in overcoming resistance. If a family is willing to perform assigned tasks, then most resistances are irrelevant and can be overcome through task assignment. Resistances such as blaming, dwelling on past injustices, and scapegoating can be directly forbidden by the therapist, and such instructions can be carried out by the more cooperative family members. The therapist may also overcome resistance by joining techniques, including minimizing demands on the family to change so that the family moves more slowly but in the desired direction.

The concept of working through, like the other concepts, is derived from psychoanalysis, but it is also quite similar to the structural concept of isomorphic transactions. It is an important concept, underscoring the need to work for an extended time with many different overt issues, all of which stem from the same dysfunctional core. Thus, in order to effect real change, a family must work a problem over and over until they have worked it through.

Modification of Family Therapy Techniques in Work with Specific Ethnic Groups

The ethnic groups described earlier, in connection with cultural influences on alcoholic family systems, also participate differently in therapy and require variations in techniques. Ethnic portraits are put forward to draw attention to common, albeit often overlooked, characteristics. They are, of course, not invariably found in every member of the group described.

The family therapy of Irish-Americans has been described in

greater detail than that of other ethnic groups. Irish-American families tend to view therapy in the same way they view confession—that is, relate sins and gain forgiveness. Yet, if the therapist uncovers their sins, they will feel embarrassed. They are not assertive and do not let the therapist know if they are inconvenienced or uncomfortable. Because of their politeness and loyalty they may comply with the therapist without really changing. They view the therapist as like a priest—as an authority whose advice must be taken seriously—and thus, will respond better to a structured, problem-oriented approach or to a specific, clearly spelled-out plan such as behavioral therapy (30). Irish families may also respond well to paradoxical techniques, which encourage change without exposing inner feelings.

Irish families rarely seek therapy on their own, so that court-mandated therapy for a substance-abusing adolescent or alcoholic father is a common reason for referral, yet embarrassing and humiliating for the family. Involving the distant father in these families is often essential to correcting the maternally dominated imbalance. Adolescent males in these families identify strongly with their fathers, although this is very difficult for them to accept. With the help of other family members, the identification with the father can be pointed out and the IP helped to reject his own extreme emotional distancing (38). Although the therapy may be very uncomfortable for these families during sessions, their deep sense of personal responsibility leads them to continue therapeutic work on their own after termination of formal therapy (30).

A key problem in the therapy of Italian-American families is the enmeshed extended family. The therapist must overcome distrust of him or her as an outsider, so that the authority necessary to change the family can be established. This may involve patiently surviving the family's many tests of the therapist's loyalty and skills. Once the therapist has gained the family's trust, the therapy can progress—for example, helping an adolescent to differentiate from the family in more adaptive ways than through substance abuse, yet permitting the young person a face-saving way to remain within the family (51).

Therapy with Italian-American families must focus on the renegotiation of their rigid system boundaries, which keep the extended family out of contact with the outside world (51). They talk openly and with exaggerated feeling, yet hide their plentiful family secrets. Secrets must be dealt with delicately, as their exposure to the therapist may constitute family betrayal (32).

Both Al-Anon and multiple-family therapy are helpful in facilitating the protection and separation of the identified patient and his or her nuclear family from the extended family of origin. With the use of an Italian co-therapist, the view of the doctor as respected can be enhanced, and other Italian families in the group who have already gone through a letting-go process may facilitate separation in still-enmeshed families (52).

Jewish-American families value credentials and education, and the therapist should not feel threatened by questions about these issues. Once credentials are established, these families readily consult with the therapist as a wise person but still retain the right to make the final judgment about which interventions they will or will not use. Many of them prefer complex, sophisticated interventions and consider behavioral types of techniques as superficial (32). Talking and expressing their feelings is often more important to Jewish-American families than actively changing, and thus they may prefer analytic techniques to strategic ones (53). However, tasks are essential in order to shift from intellectualization to action, and they can be given in the families' own complex terms, utilizing their language and rituals.

Therapists must respect the rules which support enmeshed togetherness in such families at the same time as they facilitate some essential boundary making. This can be done by working with the more flexible parts of the system, such as the adolescent subsystem. Adolescents can be encouraged to accept less threatening parental gifts while rejecting those which are infantilizing. Therapists can readily join with the children in these families, without threatening the parents, because of their basic sense of democracy and egalitarianism (53).

In white Anglo-Saxon Protestant (WASP) families, adolescent difficulties are sometimes perceived as the child's problem, not the family's (34). Thus WASP families should be encouraged to stay involved, to provide support, and to assume control of the problem. The substance-abusing adolescent should be encouraged to share his or her pain with the family so that they are moved to share the responsibility. Since asking for help may be difficult for WASP families, the therapist should support rather than confront these families in the early stages of therapy, and should build trust in order that their feelings of vulnerability will not be intensified (34). Once the problem is clearly defined and a treatment contract is made, they are likely to work hard in therapy, with the belief that this will be sufficient for success in therapy as it is in life. Thus, they respond well to educational approaches, including information about alcoholism.

In black families the constant impact of racism and discrimination is a continuing and pervasive influence which must be considered in their family therapy. Talking therapy is often not effective or acceptable in black families, particularly those that have become under-organized as a result of social pressures. In such families, structural therapy that strengthens family organization while adding to its flexibility is the most effective model.

Similar specific family patterns are seen in other ethnic groups, with relevant family interventions.

Modification of Family Therapy Techniques in Work with Families of Alcoholic Females

Because of the differences in the families of female substance abusers, family intervention strategies with women must differ from those for males. Unfortunately, relatively little research attention has been focused on the patient-treatment match for either sex. Family therapy may be more essential for female alcoholics because of their reactivity to symbolic or actual losses of spouse and children. In view of the way many female alcoholics have interacted with their fathers and husbands, one could suspect that a female therapist could achieve better rapport than a male. However, there is no evidence at this time that female therapists are more effective than male therapists with female alcoholic patients, nor that women fare any worse or better in treatment than men, despite the lack of specific techniques to meet their individual needs. In fact, female alcoholics who complete treatment are more likely than males to have a good prognosis (54).

Women substance abusers have special concerns about their children and child care. They must question how the parenting role fits into their life and establish and confirm parenting skills. Many of them have been victimized in various ways in the past, including incest, battering, and rape. Catharsis and understanding of their feelings may be essential before they can build new relationships or improve their present ties. As indicated, female substance abusers have more affective disorders than males, and these can be dealt with in a variety of ways outside of family therapy, including teaching them to deal with grief and loss, and administering appropriate antidepressant medication. However, antidepressants, particularly those with sedating effects, can be abused by substance abusers of both sexes, and they must be prescribed judiciously. It is also important that therapy not impose a stereotyped view of femininity on female patients, as this might intensify the conflicts that may have precipitated their drinking (15).

CONCLUSION

The approach described in this chapter is a synthesis of a multitude of family treatment techniques which have been used frequently over the past 25 years. A perhaps unique aspect of this approach is the synthesis of several different treatment systems that may in part seem contradictory; thus, psychodynamic techniques are advocated as well as strategic, structural, communications, systems, and behavioral methods. The use of varying techniques, depending on the unique needs of each family, stems from a commitment to individualized treatment plans. This treatment philosophy has recently influenced forms of individual therapy, even to the point where therapists do "family therapy" with only one person.

Another critical aspect of this kind of family therapy has

evolved from years of contact with recovering addict therapists and alcoholics in AA, which requires a commitment to a system for achieving abstinence. The emphasis on another system (that involving AA, Antabuse, Al-Anon, etc.), external to the system composed by the family and therapist, may seem unique to any family therapist who has not ordinarily been involved in the family's eco-system. Although many ways of achieving abstinence are frequently a part of family therapy, an emphasis on a system outside the family helps to cool down the overreactive family system.

In sum, the family therapy of alcoholic families, which has evolved from the latest quantitative family studies, sociological observations of families, and new and evolving family therapy techniques, prizes flexibility above all, valuing it above the requirements of rigid theory.

References

1. Cotton NS: The familial incidence of alcoholism. J Stud Alcohol 40:89–115, 1979

2. Lisansky ES: Alcoholism in women: social and psychological concomitants, 1: serial history data. Q J Stud Alcohol 18:588–623, 1975

3. Sherfey MJ: Psychopathology and character structure in chronic alcoholism in diet, in Etiology of Chronic Alcoholism. Edited by Helm O. Springfield, IL, Charles C Thomas, 1955

4. Bromet E, Moos R: Sex and marital status in relation to the characteristics of alcoholics. J Stud Alcohol 37:1302–1312, 1976

5. Winokur G, Clayton PJ: Family history studies, IV: comparison of male and female alcoholics. Q J Stud Alcohol 29:885–891, 1968

6. Corrigan EM: Alcoholic Women in Treatment. New York, Oxford University Press, 1980

7. Beckman LJ: Women alcoholics: a review of social and psychological studies. J Stud Alcohol 36:797–824, 1975

8. Goodwin DW, Schulsinger F, Hermansen J, et al: Alcohol problems in adoptees raised apart from alcoholic biological parents. Arch Gen Psychiatry 28:238–243, 1973

9. Roe A, Burks B: Adult adjustment of foster children of alcoholic and psychotic parentage and the influence of the foster home. Q J Stud Alcohol 6:127–141, 1945

10. Cloninger CR, Bahman M, Sigvardsson S: Inheritance of alcohol abuse. Arch Gen Psychiatry 38:861–868, 1981

11. Kaufman E, Pattison EM: Differential methods of family therapy in the treatment of alcoholism. J Stud Alcohol 42:951–971, 1981

12. Wolin S, Bennett L, Noonan D, et al: Disrupted family rituals: a factor in the intergenerational transmission of alcoholism. J Stud Alcohol 41:199–214, 1980

13. Winokur G, Cadoret R, Darzab J, et al: Depressive disease: a genetic study. Arch Gen Psychiatry 24:135–144, 1971

14. Winokur G, Cadoret R, Baker M, et al: Depressive spectrum disease versus pure depressive disease: some further data. Br J Psychiatry 127:75–77, 1975

15. Sandmaier M: The Invisible Women and Alcohol Abuse in America. New York, McGraw-Hill, 1980

16. Wilsnack SC: Alcohol abuse and alcoholism in women, in Encyclopedic Handbook of Alcoholism. Edited by Pattison EM, Kaufman E. New York, Gardner Press, 1983

17. Gomberg ES: Risk Factors Related to Alcohol Problems Among Women: Proneness and Vulnerability. Washington DC, DHEW, 1980

18. Boothroyd WE: Nature and development of alcoholism in women. In Alcohol and Drug Problems in Women. Edited by Kalant OJ. New York, Plenum Press, 1980

19. Moos RH, Finney JW, Gamble W: The process of recovery from alcoholism: comparing spouses of alcoholic patients and matched community controls. J Stud Alcohol 43:888–909, 1982

20. Edwards P, Harvey C, Whitehead PC: Wives of alcoholics: a critical review and analysis. Q J Stud Alcohol 34:112, 1973

21. Orford J, Oppenheimer E, Egert S, et al: The role of excessive drinking in alcoholism-complicated marriages: a study of stability and change over a one-year period. 12:471–495, 1977

22. Jacob T, Dunn JN, Leonard K: Patterns of alcohol abuse and family stability. Alcoholism, Clinical Experimental Research 7:382–385, 1981

23. Steinglass P: A life history model of the alcoholic family. Fam Process 19:211–226, 1980

24. Gorad SL: Communication style and interaction of alcoholics and their wives. Fam Process 10:475–489, 1971

25. Orford J, Oppenheimer E, Egert S, et al: The cohesiveness of alcoholism-complicated marriages and its influences on treatment outcome. Br J Psychiatry 128:318–319, 1976

26. Chiles JA, Strauss FS, Benjamin LS: Marital conflict and sexual dysfunction in alcoholic and nonalcoholic couples. Br J Psychiatry 173, 1980

27. Paolino TJ, McBrady BS: The Alcoholic Marriage: Alternative Perspectives. New York, Grune & Stratton, 1979

28. Billings AG, Kessler M, Gomberg CA, et al: Mutual conflict resolution of alcoholic and nonalcoholic couples during drinking and nondrinking sessions. J Stud Alcohol 40:183–195, 1979

29. Jacob T, Richey D, Evitkovic JF, et al: Communication styles of alcoholic and nonalcoholic families when drinking and not drinking. J Stud Alcohol 42:466–482, 1981

30. McGoldrick M: Irish families, in Ethnicity and Family Therapy. Edited by McGoldrick M, Pearce JK, Giordano J. New York, Guilford Press, 1982

31. Ablon J: The significance of cultural patterning for the alcoholic family. Fam Process 19:127–144, 1980

32. McGoldrick M: Normal families: an ethnic perspective, in Normal Families. Edited by Walsh F. New York, Guilford Press, 1982

33. Kaufman E: Family structures of narcotic addicts. Int J Addict 16:273–282, 1981

34. McGill D, Pearce JK: British families, in Ethnicity and Family Therapy. Edited by McGoldrick M, Pearce JK, Giordano J. New York, Guilford Press, 1982

35. Stearne MW, Pittman PJ: Alcohol abuse and the black family, in Alcohol Abuse: Black America. Edited by Harper F. Alexandria, Douglas Publishing Co., 1976

36. McLachlan JFC, Walderman RL, Birchmore DF, et al: Self-evaluation, role satisfaction, and anxiety in the woman alcoholic. Int J Addict 14:609–632, 1979

37. Schuckit M, Pitts FN, Jr, Reich T, et al: Alcoholism: two types of alcoholism in women. Arch Gen Psychiatry 20:301–306, 1969

38. Kaufman E: Substance Abuse and Family Therapy. New York, Grune & Stratton, 1985

39. Estes NJ, Baker JM: Spouses of alcoholic women, in Alcoholism: Development, Consequences, and Intervention. Edited by Estes NJ, Heinman ME. St. Louis, C.V. Mosby, 1977

40. Forrest GC: Alcoholism and Human Sexuality. Springfield, IL, Charles C Thomas, 1982

41. DHEW: Third Special Report to the U.S. Congress on Alcohol and Health. Washington, DC, U.S. Government Printing Office, 1981

42. Jackson JK: The adjustment of the family to the crisis of alcoholism. Q J Stud Alcohol 15:562–586, 1954

43. Liddle H: Five factors of failure in structural strategic family therapy: a contextual construction, in Failures in Family Therapy. Edited by Coleman S. New York, Guilford Press, 1984

44. Johnson VE: I'll Quit Tomorrow. New York, Harper & Row, 1973

45. Berenson D: The therapist's relationship with couples with an alcoholic member, in Family Therapy of Drug and Alcohol Abuse. Edited by Kaufman E, Kaufmann P. New York, Gardner Press, 1981

46. Kaufman E, Kaufmann P (eds): Family Therapy of Drug and Alcohol Abuse. New York, Gardner Press, 1979

47. Minuchin S: Families and Family Therapy. Cambridge, MA, Harvard University Press, 1974

48. Haley J: Problem-solving Therapy. San Francisco, Jossey-Bass, 1977

49. Papp P: Paradoxical strategies and countertransference, in Questions and Answers in the Practice of Family Therapy. Edited by Gurman AS. New York, Brunner-Mazel, 1981

50. Minuchin S, Fishman HC: Family Therapy Techniques. Cambridge, MA, Harvard University Press, 1981

51. Rotunno M, McGoldrick M: Italian families, in Ethnicity and Family Therapy. Edited by McGoldrick M, Pearce JK, Giordano J. New York, Guilford Press, 1982

52. Kaufman E, Borders L: Adolescent Substance Abuse in Anglo-American Families. New York, Gardner Press, 1979

53. Herz FM, Rosen EJ: Jewish families, in Ethnicity and Family Therapy. Edited by McGoldrick M, Pearce JK, Giordano J. New York, Guilford Press, 1982

54. Annis HM, Liban B: Alcoholism in women: treatment modalities and outcomes, in Alcohol and Drug Problems in Women. Edited by Kalant OJ. New York, Plenum Press, 1980

3

Issues in the Treatment of the Married Bipolar Patient: Denial and Dependency

Yolande B. Davenport, M.S.W.
Marvin L. Adland, M.D.

3

Issues in the Treatment of the Married Bipolar Patient: Denial and Dependency

We are in an era in which the biogenetic component of bipolar manic-depressive illness is generally acknowledged. Sadly, the sole treatment recommendation for this chronic familial disorder is often simple adherence to a prescribed medication regimen. Prior to the advent of psychotropic drugs (particularly lithium carbonate) that control and attenuate the disruptive mood episodes of mania and depression associated with the disorder, the course and prognosis for most bipolar patients was indeed abysmal, with long-term hospitalization often the mainstay of a limited treatment armamentarium.

But even with the best of current pharmacologic treatment, bipolar patients remain at risk for episode recurrences, psychosis, suicide, functional impairment, and disruptions in occupational, family, and social life. Furthermore, some patients discontinue their medication, causing recurrence of symptoms often severe enough to result in hospitalization; others appear to break through medication, experiencing mild to severe mood episodes; and approximately 20 percent of all diagnosed bipolar patients are reported refractory to pharmacotherapeutic intervention. Most clinical research efforts, while no longer focused upon treatment of the acute manic or depressive episode, tend to be concentrated on long-term maintenance of the patient, primarily through pharmacologic prevention methods. Drug treatment alone, however, seems scarcely sufficient to manage the intrapsychic and interpersonal distress of the patient, or reduce the burden and impact of the illness upon marriage and family. The destructive, angry, alienating, abusive behavior associated with a manic episode, and the consequences of withdrawal, helplessness, despair, and suicidal gestures and attempts associated with depression have a lasting impact upon patient, spouse, and children. In a follow-up study of bipolar patients an average of three years after hospitalization for mania, only 57 percent had been well since discharge. One-third of the patients remained functionally impaired, with moderate to severe affective symptoms (1).

The notion that euthymic periods are asymptomatic is generally not realistic.

In this chapter the focus is on a modality in which psychopharmacology and psychotherapy combined are used in the long-term maintenance of the married bipolar patient to prevent episode recurrence and to improve the quality of life for patient and family. Two psychotherapy treatment issues prominent in the maladaptive defenses observed in the manic-depressive family system, massive denial and dependency, will be discussed.

BACKGROUND

For the past 16 years at the National Institute of Mental Health (NIMH) we have treated and studied bipolar manic-depressive patients and their families in normal and pathological states. We examined psychodynamic factors associated with this familial disorder in order to understand more about the psychocultural mechanisms of transmission that may interact with genetic vulnerability in families where the disorder has occurred in at least two generations. We reported the remarkably consistent occurrence of certain themes and patterns in all of the families we studied, regardless of individual family characteristics which seem to influence the perpetuation of family pathology across generations.

We found the bipolar family system organized around massive

denial of affective feelings of loss, grief, anger, and affection, appearing as a generational repetition of failure to master early developmental issues of loss and separation in the nurturing family. When feelings are shifted from the interpersonal to more general issues, the risk of object loss is reduced, so that children observed in these families learn early that their security may rest in emotional distance. As a consequence, we noted also that strong feelings of helplessness existed in intimate and close relationships, supporting tendencies for families to remain isolated and closed from all but other family members, impeding the learning of new mechanisms for coping.

While the marriages of the couples we studied had remained intact, stresses and conflicts were seldom addressed; to do so threatened the perpetuation of the attachment, leaving both partners with a sense of vulnerability and helplessness and a fantasy that dependency supplies would be lost if anger and rage erupted. Prominent, also, among the fears noted was the possibility of recurrence of episodes, with mania viewed by the well spouse as an expression of true feelings within the control of the patient. Patients tended to blame their spouses for their illness or loss of control, as the marital relationship generally was based upon the existence of an omnipotent and omniresponsible partner who could serve as a caretaker. We have previously observed that the resistance of the couple to awareness of their dependency and their striving for independence is a major destructive pathological feature of most bipolar marriages.

Unrealistic, perfectionistic standards of conformity found in the family systems influenced the displacement of parental low self-esteem onto their children. Demands for them to succeed frequently occurred prior to an age-appropriate level of maturation, causing children to feel defective and a disappointment, replicating eventually the self-disparaging attitude of the parent. The inability of the child to achieve the perfectionism demanded by the parents revitalized fears regarding the heritable aspects of the disorder. We also noted that limits were seldom set by parents, boundaries were frequently fused, and childhood feelings of omnipotence and grandiosity were seldom thwarted. The potential patient was thus denied the experience of working through with the parent age-appropriate frustrations, a major dysfunction in the life of a child at risk for bipolar illness (2, 3). These patterns within a family constellation are not unique. We believe, however, that together with a biologic diathesis for bipolar illness, they may combine to aggravate or even precipitate overt pathology in those at risk for manic-depressive disorder.

We are fortunate to have begun our studies of bipolar couples and multigenerational families during the renewal of interest in lithium carbonate, now the drug of choice for this disorder. With the wide mood swings under control for approximately 80 percent of diagnosed patients, it was possible to engage the bipolar patient, long considered impervious to insight-oriented therapies, in psychotherapeutic efforts designed to identify, examine, and alter pathological and maladaptive behavior. We are of the opinion, however, that the powerful therapeutic effect of medication has served to keep the focus on treatment of the manic-depressive patient entirely pharmacologic. This has resulted in a paucity of attention to the persistence of psychosocial disturbance in the lives of most of these patients, including the burden the illness has placed upon marriage and family. The disorganization and chaos existent in many families is a plight which remains largely unrecognized and untreated until a crisis arises.

Because of the pernicious quality of bipolar disorder and its impact on the lives of patients, spouse, and children, we found long-term psychotherapeutic interventions essential. We advocated the inclusion of the spouse in the treatment and supported the use of psychotherapy groups of couples homogeneous for diagnosis. Our experience has convinced us that despite evidence for heritability of the disorder, psychotherapy is usually helpful and often has a decisive impact upon outcome. In a comparative study of the efficacy of couples group psychotherapy as an adjunct to lithium maintenance, we found at follow-up that patients treated in outpatient couples groups had a significantly better posthospital course than patients discharged on lithium but not assigned to a couples group (4).

In the predrug era, psychoanalysts had examined the family

constellation of the manic-depressive patient in an effort to understand etiology and elucidate treatment approaches. Freud and Abraham defined the early mother-child relationship, in which individuation and loss are first experienced and mastered, as defective in nurturing experiences in the life of the person who later develops bipolar illness. Central in their formulation of continuing problems for the person with affective disorder were loss of narcissistic input and rage at the lost object (5, 6). Jacobson perceived the interpersonal difficulties and the ego defects seen in the adult bipolar patient as related to "a particular kind of infantile narcissistic dependency"at the lost object, causing patient and partner to live in a "peculiar" "inevitably unstable" love relationship (7). Cohen et al., who focused on early cultural environment and childhood events to explain the abnormal character formation of the patient and the recurrence of the disorder in families, described an unusual and inconsistent conformity to rigid rules in the families they studied (8). Those observations were not naive with respect to the influence of biological factors in the etiology of the illness, for there was already beginning awareness of a possible biogenetic component (9, 10).

In our previous studies, we observed that failure to differentiate, massive denial in attempting to cope with distressing feelings, and generally unclear ego boundaries were among patterns transmitted from experiences in the family of origin to relationships with spouse and children. We noted that expression of affect or feeling is viewed as unsafe and that within the bipolar family system there is continuous collusion in the denial of feelings. As a result, appropriate communication of feelings is likely to be experienced as loss of control that could be destructive to dependency relationships. We perceived the defensive manuevers to avoid confrontation with conflict, observed in the bipolar marital dyad, as an unwillingness to replicate feelings of grief and rage at earlier parental losses and disappointments. In the bipolar marriage, the spouse is viewed by the patient as either the "giver" or "withholder" of gratification (2).

Over the years, our couples psychotherapy groups served us well, providing not only a modality for treatment but also a "laboratory" in which to engage in retrospective and ongoing investigations of the family system of the patient. When seven infants were born at approximately the same time to couples with at least one parent in treatment at the NIMH for bipolar disorder, we had the opportunity for prospective observation of the early nurturing attitudes and behavior of parents of infants at risk for development of a bipolar disorder. Our earlier investigations of the bipolar family system had prepared us to further test our hypotheses regarding the significance of psychocultural and psychodynamic factors in the familial occurrence and perpetuation of the disorder. We found that when mothers from bipolar families participated with their offspring in a structured laboratory playroom situation, there were differences in the children's behavior in stressful situations, and in the attitudes of these parents toward child rearing, compared with offspring and their mothers from normal control families.

By 18 months, children of bipolar parents showed less overt emotional response to separation from their mother than did normal children. The quality of the young child's attachment to the primary caretaker has been linked to the types of relationships the child is able to establish with others later. Mothers from bipolar families showed less positive feeling toward their children, and were significantly less active in interactions with them than normal control mothers. By two years of age, children with a bipolar parent had difficulty sharing with their friends and handling hostility, exhibiting measurable patterns of aggression. There were consistent differences in these children compared with normal control children, and their social and emotional problems appeared comparable to the interpersonal problems of their bipolar parents (11, 12).

The bipolar patient's responsivity to medication tends to support the likelihood of biologic abnormality in the illness, but such a constitutional factor is probably only one determinant. Developmental arrests, accessible to combinations of psychotherapeutic and pharmacologic treatment, constitute a major part of the pathology in these families, requiring in turn a major psychotherapeutic treatment effort.

Within the bipolar family system, denial serves as a major avoidance mechanism against painful feelings, and as an ego defense against the processing of distressing information. Attempts to cope with feelings of loss and grief are uncomfortable for the patient and those around him, as they provoke earlier affects, now beyond conscious awareness, regarding loss and separation and a sense that significant relationships are not dependable. Rage and feelings of helplessness reinforce the need for denial. This may precipitate withdrawal by those in the family or general environment, representing further loss or anger, perceived as further punishment by the patient. Lack of interpersonal awareness and sensitivity to affective feelings in intimate relationships results in the development of unrealistic dependency demands as well as a fear of loss of dependency supplies.

We have previously noted the preoccupation of the bipolar couple with dependency issues and our impression that patients seem to select partners who will help them defend against conscious awareness of dependency needs. The perpetuation of these maladaptive defenses may have some part in maintaining the marriages, but at a cost. Observation, investigation, and treatment of these unconscious strivings and defenses against them are ongoing therapeutic functions of our groups.

DENIAL

In previous papers, we described the massive denial of the married manic patient and its use as an adaptive defense in the interactions with the spouse (2). Enormous anxiety is provoked by a manic attack, and in a marital relationship characterized by a lack of separateness and individuation, a primitive sort of denial serves to protect both patient and spouse against awareness of loss and attendant grief. Such denial reinforces the need for strict control of affects. As we have continued to study bipolar couples and families, we have found that denial has remained a constant and persistent defensive mechanism not only for the index patients but also for their partners.

Case Example 1

In one of our couples groups, we found that all of the "well" spouses had been aware of the existence of their partners' manic-depressive disorder prior to marriage. Several had witnessed episodes of violence or were victims of violence during a manic episode. When asked about her decision to marry in spite of this knowledge, one spouse said, "Yes, I knew he had manic-depressive illness, but I did not know what it was." Yet, her husband-to-be had assaulted her—she had required plastic surgery following the assault—and he had destroyed her apartment before the police arrived and took him to the hospital. She needed to deny both awareness of the attack and her feelings about it.

Case Example 2

In the group, an index patient described at some length a quarrel at home with his wife concerning the details of a trip abroad. He accused her of procrastination and of being indecisive and overly cautious in planning the itinerary. She referred to his refusal to participate in the plans and her feeling of being in a no-win position. If she assumed the responsibility for making a unilateral decision, she was certain that should the plans not turn out well her husband would blame her. In spite of the other patients' disclaimers that their arguments were of little consequence and really did not belong in the group, members entered the discussion whole-heartedly, devoting almost the entire session to comparing their difficulties in resolving similar problems.

It was not until the session was almost over that the wife revealed that two weeks earlier she had discovered a lump on her breast and was scheduled for a biopsy the following day. When one of the therapists suggested that the husband's irritability expressed in the session was really related to concerns for his wife's well being, this was denied. The wife also joined her husband's minimization of fears regarding the pending procedure and possible results. Suggestions that both were trying to flee their pain and anxiety with diversionary minutiae pertaining to a trip were also denied. The group members, who appeared stunned by the wife's revelation, also fled their feelings.

One member commented that if the lump proved to be something serious, this was in any case an event over which there was "no control." One spouse, perhaps more in touch with reality, contributed rather sardonically, "You mean, in other words, if she dies, she dies." When adults tend to deny profound feelings and fears and find the threat of loss so difficult to tolerate, this cannot help but be transmitted in interactions with their children.

Case Example 3

In another session, a well spouse recounted an incident in which she took their 8- and 10-year-old children to meet their father at the commuter train station, as the family planned to dine together and attend an early movie. The train was very late, and when it finally arrived, the family watched husband-father, obviously angry, march past them on the platform to their car without acknowledging their presence. When one of the children asked if the father (who has a history of violent and abusive behavior) was angry, the mother replied, "No, he is not angry, he is just thinking about his work." She told the group that the children would have been frightened to learn that he was angry and, further, that they would not respect him had she answered their question truthfully, or actually confronted him. The patient subsequently said in the group that he had sat through a miserable evening, enraged and mute. Later that night, he informed his wife that he had impulsively walked out of an important meeting during the day and that he had probably lost his job.

We have previously commented on the tendency of well spouses to share many of the patients' faulty cognitions and distortions so that the spouse often does not provide the marriage with reality-based interpretations (13). In the incident above, members of the group were able to point out to the couple that an accurate interpretation for the children of the father's mood might have been less frightening than their possible fantasies regarding the source of his anger and possible fears of retaliation. It is a disservice in the early life of a child at risk for manic-depressive illness when parents fail to permit the child opportunities to experience and endure pain and disappointment.

While denial is a ubiquitous mental mechanism used by almost everyone at some time, in our view it is not a "primary" mechanism. Rather, it is a mechanism of response, and a defense against the mounting anxiety that occurs when expression and gratification of needs and drives are frustrated. In our observations of bipolar patients with their children, we have seen that feelings of both dependence and assertiveness have no room for expression and are suppressed by both the patient and surrounding family members. The taboo in the family against recognition and statement of needs and feelings is immense, so that resolution of important life-long issues is seldom achieved. The faulty but basic formula in the bipolar system appears to be that if feelings are expressed, abandonment and rejection will follow. We have seen this in operation especially around issues involving conflicts of dependence.

DEPENDENCY

The husband and wife in any family system bring the themes and patterns of their respective families of origin to a new relationship, transmitting similar themes to successive generations. Provocativeness in the relationship of the married bipolar couple stems largely from unresolved dependency issues and fears of object loss that predate the marriage. Where the marriage of the bipolar patient has remained intact, the needs and mutual dependency of the couple appear to be the binding factors that serve to perpetuate the relationship (14). A consistent recurring theme throughout our group sessions revolved around infantile dependency demands and the interdependence the couples have around very primitive needs.

In the bipolar marriage there always seems to be a need to have one spouse in the dependent position. A recurrent question in the relationship is often who will cater to whose infantilism. In infantile character organization there is a hypersensitivity to any impending or occurring frustration. Needs are to be fulfilled even when the demand is not articulated. When there is a delay in fulfilling a demand or if the demand is impossible to fulfill, the bipolar patient bypasses the feelings of loss and sadness and instead immediately shifts into an escalating rage. This rage proceeds further from one specific issue to encompass a general condemnation of the "depriving" person. When the demand is unfulfilled and the infantile wish of the patient is thwarted, anxiety arises. Understanding and interpreting the meaning of unbearable emotional pain is a function the couples group is often able to perform for its members.

Case Example 4

John, the index patient, announced shortly after arrival at a group session that on a scale of 0–10 he felt his wife rated a "4" in mania. Mary, startled, was silent. Challenged by the group, John said that Mary was irritable and on the way to the session had nearly hit an elderly woman pedestrian in the crosswalk. Mary denied her husband's allegations, stating she was perfectly aware of the pedestrian. John then expounded at length on "the right" of pedestrians, and how vulnerable he felt in that position. He thought his wife overly preoccupied with "things other than safe driving," and explained at length to the group that she was heavily invested in a job-related project, and he added sarcastically that in her job she earned less than $8,000 annually. Mary quietly explained that the project had been finished two weeks ago. John's voice then began to escalate as he described how Mary never cleaned the stove top after cooking, and how their refrigerator had broken down one week ago and he had had to phone for the repairman. It was clear that he felt his wife had failed to perform what he considered to be her proper functions. But even worse—and his voice became quite shrill—Mary had failed to stop at the grocery several nights in succession and now there was no skim milk in the refrigerator, and there were no bananas. He suggested gratuitously that Mary could not add or she would have noted the last time she bought bananas that she had not bought enough for the week.

It seemed as if John, a lawyer who surely knew the direction to the closest grocery, thought he would starve without his wife's caretaking. He appeared threatened by a realization of Mary's growing determination in their relationship to begin to attend to her own needs. Further, he related that things had been going badly for him at his firm—his boss was a "machine"—and since his wife was busy with her activities and had not been home for several evenings, he had been unable to discuss his problems with her. Not, he added, that his wife could help him constructively with any decisions regarding his work. During this tirade, Mary looked nonplussed. Her strivings toward independence had provoked envy and rage in John, causing him to feel threatened and vulnerable.

Another index patient in the group, Michael, said that everyone knew from past history that whenever John referred to the meagerness of his wife's salary, this was a signal that John was hypomanic. Referring to John's stressful work situation and his attack on Mary, Michael further remarked on the need of the bipolar patient to be able to blame someone when disappointing or hurtful events occurred. He said, "Someone has to be blamed; when I am hypomanic I also blame my wife, but mostly I am now able to blame myself." Then with amusement he added, "However, since I inherited that need-to-blame trait from my mother, I really blame her."

"No milk in the refrigerator" and "no bananas" became key words for the group long after that session. They seemed to represent for all of the couples the problems each shared in resolving dependency issues and reaching reasonable resolutions. For some time, the group used the session for further discussion of the rage John felt around his unmet needs, his unrealistic fears of helplessness, his belief that his wife was the sole medium of his happiness, and his inability to understand that he was truly capable of accepting responsibility for replenishment of supplies.

Case Example 5

Another instance of not dealing with conflictual dependency needs occurred in one of our groups when the cotherapist, an object of much sincere affection by the members, was frequently absent without explanation. There were fantasies that he might accept a promotion which would take him away from the group. At each session his absence would be discussed and lamented, but no angry feelings could be elicited. Instead, there were amused interpretations regarding the irritable feelings of the remaining therapist, amidst assurances that little significance should be attached to the absent therapist since "You're here—you run the sessions anyhow." When the absent therapist at last reappeared, the group seemed relieved. One group member, fearing that the therapist might react to any suggestions of hostility, hastily mollified by commenting, "Even though you have missed too many sessions, we love you just the same." It was as if they were caught up in some delusional belief of their total dependence for survival on one they viewed both as irreplaceable and as vulnerable to an angry assault from them. When in time the therapist predictably began to falter even more, and it was demonstrably evident that he was no longer available for their care, the group began to settle down to understand and interpret their sense of vulnerability.

It was as if they were experiencing a replication of what had happened in their own families when they were young and could not protest or express anger, fearing rejection and the sense of loss and emptiness which might follow. Confronting the maladaptive beliefs and teaching patients to link provoking incidents or urges to both their repressed feelings and their catastrophic emotional responses is an important therapeutic task. The examples we cited are really two sides of the same coin; in both, immobilization occurred because of unreasonable dependency demands.

DENIAL AND DEPENDENCY ISSUES IN BIPOLAR CHILD-REARING ATTITUDES

Earlier in this chapter, we referred to studies of children of bipolar parents performed at the NIMH and to preliminary findings. During simulated test situations conducted when the children were 12, 15, and 18 months of age, we became increasingly aware of how the intrapsychic defenses of the infants in bipolar families come to be mobilized at a very early age. To illustrate, when appointments were made for visits to the laboratory playroom, the mothers were routinely informed that each visit would last two hours. In contrast to behavior of normal control mothers, who traveled with the usual infant care paraphernalia, bipolar mothers were more likely to come from home without the necessary equipment. During the third round of sessions, when the infants were able to ask for cookies or crackers, there were still index mothers unable to produce these comforting items. This phenomenon by no means implies that these mothers disliked or rejected their children. Rather, it may represent a serious cognitive defect in their understanding of the relationship between the time required for the testing situation and the basic dependency needs of their infants; or quite simply, the inability to ask themselves the natural question, "What do I need to do or bring in order to care for my child?" A child exposed to this kind of defect from the primary caretaker so early in the nurturing stage must come to feel that it is unsafe to rely on anyone, and consequently may grow up with an exaggerated denial of dependence and counterdependency behaviors evolving from this awareness.

The following is excerpted from process notes from one videotaped test episode.

Case Example 6

A mother arrived early and sat in the hallway with her 15-month-old infant balanced precariously on her knee at a distance from her body. The child was charming and babbled ingratiatingly without fear to anyone who stopped to talk to him. The mother's affect was depressed and anxious. When the child became restless during the wait, one of the staff members produced a toy to amuse him, as the mother had brought none. It seemed a clear message to the child that his mother was unable to provide for his needs and that he must look elsewhere. In the bipolar family the dilemma becomes even greater at times when the need to turn to someone outside for gratification is very likely to be interfered with by the family.

In the playroom, mother and child were alone initially. She deposited him on the floor in a position where his right leg was caught behind him. Although he whimpered, he remained so until a staff member entered the room to free him. When procedures for the paradigm were discussed, she was informed about a "free play" period with her child. She then asked for more detail, commenting, "I don't play with him." When his nose began to run, the mother reached for her pocketbook, which had no tissues. Still later, when the mother left the room as planned, the child ignored her departure and rapidly engaged with "the stranger" who had entered according to plan. On observing the child's apparently easy acceptance of the separation, the mother commented behind the one-way mirror, "He doesn't even miss me."

The mother's history is also one of considerable deprivation, for she was abandoned by her parents at age five and lived in numerous foster homes until her marriage. This child's adaptation reflected his early nurturing experience. Shortly after coming home from the hospital with the newborn child, his parents enforced an early rejection of his discomfort, tuning out his crying by turning up their stereo speakers and placing his bassinet between them so that he could not be heard. Crying as a positive communication of feelings depends upon an appropriate response. When not attended to, the child may resort to the defense of denial of feelings of dependency.

In a recent paper, we described how new bipolar parents in the NIMH study encouraged their children to leave the dependency stage too quickly. We have speculated that this may represent the parents' need for reassurance that their child is "ready," on a par at least with other children, but often in advance of the appropriate maturational stage (11). Perhaps this sustains their belief that if the child does all right, they too are all right, and it is less necessary to fear their own inadequacies as well as the possible genetic endowment. We have also observed how the inconsistency and variableness in the moods of bipolar parents may deprive the child of a consistent and available source of nurturance. Two of the children who were seen in the laboratory at times when their mothers were depressed appeared significantly aware of the mothers' moods. They were observed in attempts to comfort them; this was interpreted as not necessarily representative of the children's altruism but as attempts to defend against the overwhelming anxiety produced by the mothers' withdrawal during their depression. One must also consider the significance of the burden imposed upon a child who must comfort his mother at an age when the roles should be reversed.

In the bipolar family, a child learns at an early age to maintain control over affective reaction, whether sadness, disappointment, anxiety, or anger. The opportunity to experience and endure pain seldom occurs when the goal is to avoid and flee those feelings. Because of inconsistency of parental behavior, the child never knows what will happen or whether his needs will be met, and must come to believe he is always in a dangerous situation.

Lacking the developmental experience of learning to recognize feelings leads to a life-long deficit in the ability to translate and communicate an awareness of feelings to the self and others.

We saw the children in the laboratory at an interval in their development when the sense of oneness with the mother was changing. Children from normal control families expressed distress in the separation sequences by crying and acknowledging the pain of loss. Though the expression of pain is the appropriate affect, this affect may be repressed or denied because it awakens further distancing by the mother as she responds to her own inner discomfort. The infant is faced with a double loss: first, the immediate separation from the parent, and second, the accelerated distancing that may come if the child protests. The infant quickly learns that the initial loss must be denied and the affects around it repressed. One way for this to manifest itself is through diverting attention from the loss that has occurred. We are then viewing a childhood conditioning experience resulting in a pattern of behavior in dependent relationships which becomes the template for feeling (nonfeeling) and behavior in future adult relationships. What happened in the vignette described above may seem relatively unimportant, but our experience suggests that this may be an example of a precursor to the coping mechanisms adapted by the adult bipolar patient, which grow with time, encompassing most relationships.

Within the marital relationship of the bipolar patient, the dependency needs, wants, and drives of the couple become subverted, since each spouse has a quality that says that it must be the other who gives. There are, of course, constructive aspects of dependency, but so often in the bipolar dyad and the bipolar family, one sees only the exploitation of dependency.

MULTIPLE FAMILY GROUP THERAPY

Although we are aware of the biogenetic factors predisposing to overt bipolar illness, manifestations of the disorder do not occur in a psychosocial vacuum. The gross pathological behavior of the bipolar patient that was associated with the disorder in the past is now often less evident because of the effects of medication. Fewer patients and their families may now seek help for the underlying maladaptive attachment behaviors and defects in emotional regulation associated with the illness. However, we believe that it is highly important that these patients know that they can return to the therapist for emotional support and nurturance even after discharge. When treated with medication to relieve severe rapid mood swings, the bipolar patient is better able to work in psychotherapy, to alter and change maladaptive defenses, and to improve communication patterns. The denial and opaqueness which seem to much a part of the personality of the bipolar patient constitute a powerful defense. There is no quick or easy resolution; brief psychotherapeutic intervention seldom has lasting or meaningful effects.

We have strongly supported the need for continuity and consistency in treatment in our work with bipolar couples and families. A study completed in two of our lithium clinics at the NIMH found that patients on medication seen with their wives for treatment in our open-ended groups received better scores at follow-up on two parameters (adherence to medication and compliance with appointment keeping) (15). As therapists, it is possible we have become overly concerned about the dependency needs of our patients, perhaps because of our own anxieties around dependency as a countertransference issue. Nevertheless, we believe that these couples, particularly those who are parents, need to be seen regularly if the psychopathology that is multigenerationally engrained and pervasive is to be interrupted.

New awareness and new insights are possible in a therapeutic program such as the couples group, which introduces and permits experimentation with new ways of being. We also believe that it is possible to alter the emotional and developmental course of the offspring of bipolar patients (children at risk) by intervening in the perpetuation of faulty parenting patterns. In our experience listening to these patients and their family members in groups, conjointly, and in individual sessions, we have learned how early in their psychological evolution they became exposed to anxiety and an unending struggle around issues of dependence-independence, separation, and loss. They are stunted in their ability to grieve, to mourn a loss and to carry on. With the burden of a genetic predisposition to bipolar illness, these patients live a life focused on the half-empty glass, always anticipating that it will become emptier still. To refer to two of our earlier vignettes, no matter how much Mary contributed to the marriage and family—working, keeping house, raising their five children almost single-handedly because of her husband's ups and downs—for John it was not enough. On the other hand, in the absent therapist vignette, the group members were so frozen and immobilized by the loss of an important "family" member that they were unable to notice that the glass was already empty and that there was an alternative to their loss. This is a recurrent long-term illness with lasting effects; the therapeutic task is fiercesome at best.

Continuity of the psychotherapy is essential in the treatment, and a therapeutic alliance which adds stability to the inconsistent behavior associated with this episodic disorder is required for a long time. Our ideas about treatment are in sharp contrast to the current common practice of pharmacologic intervention alone. The couples groups we described lasted for many years without any preselection for "best results." We have previously noted the specific therapeutic advantages that the couples psychotherapy group modality provides: 1) spouse involvement counteracts patient efforts to distort, deny, and flee treatment; 2) the initial diffusion of transference reduces anxiety about intimacy and closeness; 3) a supportive group copes with fears about the genetic component of the illness; 4) mutual sensitivity results in early warnings from the group, permitting earlier drug and psychotherapeutic intervention; and 5) group cohesiveness with a common denominator of affective illness supports the thrusts toward socially desirable behavior, including adherence to a prescribed medication regimen (4,15). The therapeutic task of the group is primarily one of intervention, interpretation, and reeducation. Effective therapeutic intervention, and any long-term psychotherapy with bipolar patients, may require more than one treating person—no one person can long withstand the assault. There must be a treatment team (we have used the co-therapist model with weekly support from a psychoanalyst consultant), and there must be a willingness for someone on that team to be available at all times. Serious deprivations in early developmental periods leave these patients with a massive sensitivity to signs of possible loss. This in turn leads to massive reaction and overreaction, at times of panic proportions. Bipolar patients and their families require a long and intense interaction with therapists and treating institutions before they develop a therapeutic alliance in which they can gradually view life's glass as half full rather than half empty. In time, this will lead them to find strength in themselves and confidence in their own capacity to refill the glass.

We have seen the effectiveness of our therapeutic model. It does work, and we believe that replication will produce results like ours—a positive effect on this enormous public health problem.

References

1. Carlson GA, Kolin J, Davenport YB, et al: Follow-up of 53 bipolar manic depressive patients. Br J Psychiatry 124:134–139, 1974

2. Ablon SL, Davenport YB, Gershon ES, et al: The married manic. Am J Orthopsychiatry 45:854–866, 1975

3. Davenport YB, Adland ML, Gold PW, et al: Manic-depressive illness: psychodynamic features of multigenerational families. Am J Orthopsychiatry 49:24–35, 1979

4. Davenport YB, Ebert MH, Adland ML, et al: Couples group therapy as an adjunct to lithium maintenance of the manic patient. Am J Orthopsychiatry 47:495–502, 1977

5. Freud S: Mourning and Melancholia (1917), in Collected Papers, vol. 4. Edited by Jones E. London, Hogarth Press, 1956

6. Abraham K: Notes on the psychoanalytical investigation and treatment of manic-depressive insanity and allied conditions, in Selected Papers on Psychoanalysis. London, Hogarth Press, 1949

7. Jacobson E: Interaction between psychotic partners, I: Manic-depressive partners, in Neurotic Interaction in Marriage. Edited by Eisenstein VW. New York, John Wiley, 1956

8. Cohen MB, Baker G, Cohen RA, et al: An intensive study of 12 cases of manic-depressive psychosis. Psychiatry 17:103–137, 1954

9. Kraepelin E: Manic-depressive Insanity and Paranoia. Translated by Barclay M. Edinburgh, ES Livingston, 1921

10. Werthem FL: A group of benign chronic psychoses: prolonged manic excitements. Am J Psychiatry 9:17–78, 1920

11. Davenport YB, Zahn-Waxler C, Adland ML, et al: Early child-rearing practices in families with a manic-depressive parent. Am J Psychiatry 141:230–235, 1984

12. Zahn-Waxler C, McKnew D, Cummings M, et al: Problem behaviors and peer interactions of young children with manic-depressive behavior. AM J Psychiatry 141:236–240, 1984

13. Dibble ED, Davenport YB, Guroff JJ: Maladaptive attitudes of manic-depressive patients and their spouses: measurements and therapeutic implications. Presented at the Annual Meeting of the American Orthopsychiatry Association, Washington, DC, 1979

14. Davenport YB: Treatment of the married bipolar patient in conjoint couples psychotherapy groups, in Family Therapy and Major Psychopathology. Edited by Lansky MR. New York, Grune & Stratton, 1981

15. Connelly CE, Davenport YB, Nurnberger JI: Adherence to treatment regimen in a lithium carbonate clinic. Arch Gen Psychiatry 30:585–588, 1982

4

Involving Families in Treating Schizophrenia: The Role of Family Education

Kathryn L. West, Ph.D.
Louis Cozolino, Ph.D.
Barnet Malin, M.D.
Geneva G. McVey, R.N., C.
Melvin R. Lansky, M.D.
Carol R. Bley, M.S.W.

4

Involving Families in Treating Schizophrenia: The Role of Family Education

In 1983 the Family Treatment Program at the Brentwood Hospital instituted a formal program of education for the families of schizophrenic patients. A careful review of the literature had encouraged us to add this component to the already well-established, family-oriented treatment program that characterized the unit. The experiences of others who have developed and studied family education programs enabled us to anticipate problems and devise an educational component that could be fully integrated into the existing treatment program.

The present report is intended to provide others with guidelines for developing family education in treatment settings similar to ours. Although our program is relatively new and we are not yet in a position to fully assess its effectiveness, we judge it to have value. It is our clinical experience that the education program has contributed significantly to the treatment of patients and to the development of a helpful, collaborative relationship with our patients' families.

In recent years, diverse factors have led to a revival of interest in the relationship between family interactions and schizophrenia. First, the characteristic pattern of community-based care for schizophrenic patients includes a relatively brief inpatient period followed by extended aftercare in the community. Adequate transitional living environments are rare, and patients who in the past would have faced long periods of hospitalization often return to their families in states of partial remission. Examinations of these family environments and the problems resulting from the return home of a disturbed and disturbing relative have revealed that this posthospital period is often one of intense stress for the entire family system. Second, the work by Brown and colleagues (1) and later by Vaughn and Leff (2) in Great Britain provided empirical evidence that deleterious aspects of the family environment could be specified and measured with standardized procedures. Their work on *expressed emotion* (EE), which was assumed to reflect ongoing intrafamilial attitudes and processes, suggested that the schizophrenic patient was particularly sensitive to certain discriminable attributes of the family emotional environment. An awareness that family members are increasingly responsible for the aftercare of a schizophrenic relative and that specific attributes of the family environment may be particularly noxious has led to renewed interest in family intervention programs designed to prevent relapse and foster social recovery.

At the same time, growing consumerism and antipsychiatry sentiment have led relatives to seek more information about mental illness and the adequacy and appropriateness of the treatment their family members are receiving. Information appears to be of critical importance for the family during the initial crisis, and the need continues throughout the period of recovery. The inclusion of at least an initial phase of family education in a treatment program seems warranted.

Educating families of psychiatric patients is a relatively new movement, and systematic assessments of the effects of psychoeducational programs have not yet been done. Thus far, the effectiveness of family education has been measured primarily through open-ended information tests designed to assess the acquisition of information by the relatives.

A recent study by Berkowitz and her colleagues (3) attempted to assess the results of a four-session educational component at the beginning of their long-term treatment program (4). Pre- and posttests were given to both experimental (educated) and control groups, with an approximate six-week interval before beginning long-term treatment. At the six-week follow-up, relatives who had received the education were more knowledgeable about the diagnosis than those in the control group. Follow-up measures also showed a significant difference between the subgroups of high EE relatives within each of the two conditions. Those who received education had a greater knowledge of recommended management procedures and had a higher degree of optimism about the patient's future. The low EE relatives in the two conditions did not differ. In discussing these findings, Berkowitz and her colleagues suggest a differential impact on families rated as high and low in expressed emotion. Since the education is attempting to teach "low EE-type" attitudes, it may be that high EE relatives are able to show statistically significant changes while low EE relatives already have more therapeutic attitudes and have fewer changes to make. It may also be that the different styles with which high EE and low EE families interact and cope are what cause the differences in learning patterns.

Snyder and Liberman (5) reported using four outcome measures for family education. A knowledge questionnaire that was given to relatives before and after the two-session educational program showed an increase of from 40 percent to 80 percent in correct answers. A six-month follow-up with the Camberwell Family Interview showed that with family education and therapy two-thirds of the high EE relatives became low EE, while without the family education and therapy, only one-third of the high EE control subjects became low EE. Further, at the six-month follow-up, positive effects of the total program were found in a measure of perceived conflictual situations and in satisfaction ratings. These measures cannot be interpreted as outcome measures for family education alone because of the addition of a treatment component.

In another study, a semi-structured consumer satisfaction interview was conducted at the homes of 10 families who had gone through family education without being involved in any form of treatment (6). The education program was based on those designed by the Falloon (7) and Anderson (8) groups and was geared to address issues of concern to the relatives of young first-break patients. The data from these family interviews suggest specific and nonspecific effects of family education and raise many possibilities for investigating the effectiveness and possible drawbacks of presenting family education without treatment.

Over all, the relatives who were interviewed found that most of the theoretical information was interesting but too general to be of much practical use. The exception was information concerning the medication and its side effects. Relatives seemed to be most appreciative of practical management advice, at least during the initial phase of the patient's reintegration into the home and community. The sessions seemed to have the positive effect of reducing the families' anxieties about the acute illness and creating the feeling of a lifeline between the families and the treatment program. Relatives also reported feeling a greater degree of encouragement to keep their relative on medication as a result of the sessions.

In general, relatives were not disturbed by the information they received, except for families who had expected the patient to show a rapid recovery and who learned that a recovery period of one to two years was likely if the patient was experiencing the acute stage of the illness. The possibility of a chronic, lifetime prognosis was not addressed with these families of first-break patients. Relatives found the information pitched at the proper level and were particularly impressed by biochemical explanations of neural transmission and the effects of medication. Only one out of ten relatives thus far has been willing to participate in a family support group. This points to the existence of a large population of relatives of the mentally ill who are not participating in relatives' groups and thus may not be represented in studies directed toward assessing family needs for education (9, 10).

In the area of information, relatives stressed the priority of specific management over theoretical information. At least initially, survival skills superseded curiosity in their minds. The more concrete the information, and the more it related specifically to the patient, the more useful it was. Relatives reported great difficulty in translating general advice into specific behaviors at home. Unsuccessful attempts to implement advice appeared to produce discouragement and an increase in feelings of pessimism and guilt. Parents reported concern about the possibility that their other children would become ill, and requested more information in this area. Further research may show that equipping relatives with survival skills should have priority over and precede the presentation of general information, especially when educational programs are conducted without family therapy.

The consensus regarding format was that follow-up and feedback are essential, especially in the implementation of management advice. Relatives suggested that the information be given slowly, repeatedly, and simply, especially at first. When the sessions were spread out over time there was a better opportunity to implement and monitor the effects of specific management tips and to receive feedback. Relatives also reported changes in symptoms over the course of treatment and expressed their need for updated advice as new difficulties arose. The reports from families suggested that given limited resources, a slowly paced educational program with long intervals between sessions is preferable to a concentrated program that is given when the patient is first released from the hospital.

These findings suggest that family education in the absence of ongoing support would be far from adequate, for there would be no way in which to assess how the educational information was interpreted and utilized. This underscores the value of having an educational program closely integrated into a family treatment program that spans the entire period of patient treatment, from the onset of hospitalization through aftercare; such a treatment program can provide families with the ongoing support and psychotherapy they require in addition to education. The material that follows presents our experience with the integration of an educational component into a family treatment program for schizophrenic patients and their families.

THE PLACE OF EDUCATION IN THE BRENTWOOD FAMILY TREATMENT PROGRAM

When the Family Treatment Program at the Brentwood Hospital instituted the program of education for the families of the schizophrenic patients on the unit, the rationale for adding an educational component came not only from the experience of others with such programs, as reported above, but also from the clinical experience of the unit's staff. The staff supported the opinion that it would be beneficial to our patients and their families to have an in-house forum for presenting information about schizophrenia in a systematic way, consistent with the philosophy of the treatment program.

The Family Treatment Program is part of the total treatment of all patients, including those who bear the diagnosis of schizophrenia, on an inpatient psychiatric unit with a well-developed psychosocial orientation. In addition to providing patients with general psychiatric care, the Family Treatment Program offers individual and group psychotherapies and specializes in involving the family and friends of the schizophrenic patient in the treatment.

The unit endeavors to maximize the benefits of treatment for the patient, to meet the needs of the patient's social support system outside the hospital, and to establish a collaborative program of care that will minimize the need for rehospitalization. We have been able to identify some family attributes that may either contribute to or interfere with the patient's successful response to treatment, and we attempt to use this knowledge to help the patient's family undergo beneficial attitudinal and behavioral changes. The established modalities of family treatment have been family therapy and multiple family therapy.

As professionals working with schizophrenic patients, the treatment staff had become increasingly aware of the need for educating relatives about the illness. Prior to the formal program, education had been carried out primarily in an informal way, in the contexts of treatment planning, psychodynamic family therapies, and aftercare planning. Inevitably there was redundancy and inconsistency in the delivery of factual information to the patient's family. The introduction of a structured educational component to the unit's treatment program was conceived of as a necessary, more effective way of disseminating informational material that would help the patient and his or her family understand the illness and reduce the emotional turbulence that results from ignorance or from a refusal to acknowledge the presence of an illness.

The education program addresses the definition of schizophrenia, describes positive and negative symptoms and other phenomena related to the illness, presents theories about its etiology and prognosis, teaches basic scientific information about the brain and its functioning, explains the relevance of different aspects of treatment, and provides a forum in which families can ask questions and make use of the knowledge and experience of the treatment staff in order to satisfy their need to know.

Families participate in the education program as soon as possible after the patient has been hospitalized. The group setting for providing information about the illness is seen as an initial step in the ongoing treatment and continuing education of the patient and his relatives. It serves as a focused, specialized form of intervention that plays a specific role—organizing and orienting as well as educational—in the integrated, overall treatment regimen of the unit. Its primary intent is to serve as an informational basis for understanding schizophrenia, which will facilitate and enhance the further learning that relatives will experience as they participate in the different modalities of family therapy provided for them.

In the family psychotherapy that families receive, there is an opportunity for them to address their own particular needs and problems. In this setting, participants acquire an understanding of how the illness affects their family unit. As they explore the impact of the illness upon them as individuals and as a family group, their knowledge about schizophrenia will take on new and meaningful dimensions.

In multiple family therapy, several families with a schizophrenic member meet with each other, and family members have the opportunity to identify with their counterparts in other families, to learn from the experiences other families have had, and to provide valuable support for one another. Their understanding of the illness and the accompanying interpersonal vulnerabilities increases as they discover how these are manifested in other patients and how others have learned to cope with their consequences.

The incorporation of an educational component into an established, highly functional treatment unit has required careful thought and planning by the unit staff. It has been necessary to be clear in our understanding of what role the education should play so that it could be integrated with and complementary to the treatment goals of the unit.

In describing the education component that has been developed by the Brentwood Family Treatment Program, we shall focus on issues that require special consideration by the staff of any unit interested in incorporating education into its overall regimen of treatment. The issues include selection of the informational content, presentation of the material, and management of the education program.

The Selection of Informational Content

The range, diversity, and nature of the content to be included in an educational program will depend primarily on the treatment philosophy and particular interventions of the unit into which the education is being introduced. On a treatment unit where opinions about the diagnosis, etiology, and treatment of schizophrenia may vary widely, the staff must first identify their own areas of agreement, on which they can then base a program of education for families. Decisions about what to include may be made on the basis of the staff's clinical experience and their understanding of what information has been found to be most effective.

Selecting information content for its educational program was not a problem for the Family Treatment Program, which has a long history and a focused treatment philosophy. On our unit an effort is constantly made to identify both those aspects of each case that reflect biological vulnerability for psychosis and those that represent a psychosocial attempt at protection from such vulnerability. The staff recognizes the complexity of the illness and endeavors to communicate that to the patients and their families. A major message we impart, for example, is that relatives *do not cause* schizophrenia but relatives *can be of great help* in the recovery process. Making it clear to family members that the staff does not hold them responsible for or blame them for the illness can be an important initial step in building a therapeutic alliance that will enable collaboration between family and staff rather than accentuate the defensiveness of the patient's relatives. This in turn serves as a model for collaboration between the family and the patient that can replace family patterns of blame and guilt.

A related issue that requires discussion by a staff is whether it is better to present information to families as fact or as opinion. Ultimately, the degree of certainty with which informational data are presented becomes a matter of clinical judgment based on the staff's goals and experience and on the particular group of patients and relatives participating. In our presentation of information, the staff of the Family Treatment Program makes an effort to separate fact from opinion and to identify clearly which is which. For example, in discussing the biological and neurophysiological aspects of schizophrenia, the psychiatrist describes the transmission of information through the dopamine system "as best we understand it." We openly acknowledge the continuing mysteries that surround the illness of schizophrenia, and our experience has been that both patients and families can accept and respect scientific uncertainty.

The Presentation of Educational Material

The Brentwood Family Treatment Program staff presents its education program in one session of approximately two hours, as follows:

1:00 p.m. Introduction to Family Education
Chief Psychiatrist
1:15 p.m. Diagnosis and Symptoms
Clinical Psychologist
1:45 p.m. Biology, Neurophysiology, and Pharmacology
Psychiatry Resident
2:30 p.m. The Family and Social Factors
Head Nurse and/or Senior Social Worker

The schedule allows time for questions and answers after each presentation.

As indicated, the education program is staffed by members of the different professional groups working on the unit. This has several advantages, including providing families with an opportunity to meet different members of the treatment team and observe the collaborative nature of their presentations.

Two sections of the education program are presented by physicians: the introduction, by the psychiatrist who is in charge of the ward; and the section dealing with biological material, by the psychiatry resident. Our decision to use medical staff for both of these presentations was based on data from the family interviews cited above (6), which revealed that the presence of a medical doctor inspires confidence in the families who participate. Not only is it appropriate for a physician to present the medical material but also having a physician explain and support the roles of other professions apparently helps relatives accept the concept that treatment involves more than medication and psychological and psychosocial forms of intervention are legitimate and valuable.

In general, the selection of individuals to be responsible for the different components of the education must depend upon the interest and competence of professional persons available for the tasks. In our experience, if two or more different staff members can share the responsibility for presenting each of the education sections, they can cover for each other when one of them is unavailable. We have also found that trainees assigned to the ward (psychiatry residents, psychology interns, and social work interns) often are interested in the education program and can be trained to participate in the presentations. It is possible, as well, to use audio or audio-visual aids as a substitute for a presentation by a staff member. Should this be necessary for the biochemical section of the program, however, it is important to have a staff member present who is familiar with the basics of neuroanatomy and the hypothesized action of the antipsychotic medications and who can discuss the material and respond to the questions that inevitably arise.

The Management of the Education Program

Coordination. We have found it important to have at least one staff person responsible for the overall management of the program. This individual is committed to remain throughout the entire session, to greet relatives, to administer any research measures that may be wanted, to distribute printed materials, and generally to provide a sense of continuity. Having one person serve in this capacity makes it easier for other staff members to rotate through the program, overlapping only briefly, to make their presentations and respond to questions.

Number of sessions. Our education program takes place in a single session, but it is presented in the context of an ongoing treatment program which provides relatives with the opportunity to integrate the information they have received, to ask questions, and to discuss problems further with the treatment staff. Thus, our program differs from some of the educational programs described in the clinical research studies cited above, which have several sessions instead of only one. Multiple sessions would be an alternative way of providing for integration and feedback.

Timing the education. We make an effort to have families receive education early in the patient's hospitalization. However, the scheduling of any given family for the education program is a staff decision based on our assessment of when the relatives will achieve maximum benefit from the experience. In most cases, a family's attendance at an education program is determined by the willingness of the relatives to participate and their having the time to do so.

Intuitively, it might seem that relatives need the information the program can offer as close to the onset of the patient's illness as possible. However, in our experience families seek information and find it most meaningful only when they are ready to hear it. The family may not be ready to face the fact that the patient has a serious illness until the patient has had two or three psychotic episodes. This is particularly true of families who react to the patient's psychosis as if it were a variant of normal willfulness rather than a psychiatric illness. When this occurs, the family's response to the patient is almost certain to be hostile and unsympathetic. Such families change their attitudes and alter their behaviors only with great difficulty and emotional pain.

The concerns of families and the questions relatives ask seem to differ according to the phase of the illness. During the acute period, while the patient is in the hospital, their concern usually focuses on the positive symptoms (that is, hallucinations and delusions) of the illness, and they attempt to make sense of the behavior that brought the patient to the hospital. Later, when the patient's symptoms are in remission and he or she is ready for discharge from the hospital, relatives seek management advice and strategies for coping with the patient in the home and community. Issues relating to the long-term care of the patient are a major concern to families, even when the remission is excellent and the circumstances of the family are emotionally benign.

A treatment program that provides both inpatient and outpatient care can serve both sets of needs in its education component.

The consumers of family education. The education program is open to any member of the patient's immediate or extended family and to close friends, as well. Those who participate are essentially self-selected, which increases the likelihood that their participation is appropriate. The closeness of the relationship between the patient and the other person or persons is one factor that determines attendance. However, in our experience, relatives who are more detached, such as an adult sibling, may also attend in an effort to understand the illness for their own sake.

The number of relatives and friends present at any one education session affects the atmosphere of the meeting and determines the amount of time available in which individuals can ask questions. Two or three families (approximately six to nine persons) constitute a small enough group to offer an intimate environment in which those present feel comfortable sharing common experiences. Such interactions between individuals add an important element of support to the process of the group. Larger sessions tend to take on a less personal quality and a more didactic tone, and there are fewer interactions among those present. In a larger group, families tend to ask fewer questions, especially questions that involve personal details about their ill relative. The staff must consider both the goals of the program and the staff resources when deciding how many families are to be involved.

Supplementary educational materials. We have found that different kinds of handouts play an important role in an education program. For example, it is helpful for participants to have copies of whatever visual aids are used to illustrate the educational material. We distribute a diagram of a synapse to illustrate how medication is involved. We also provide printed materials giving information about community resources and family support groups. Other helpful items include a chart showing ward personnel and a list of staff telephone numbers.

If it is necessary for any of the presentations to be made on audiotape rather than in person, it is especially important to provide participants with transcriptions of the presentation. It is sometimes difficult to follow such tapes in the absence of a speaker, and the transcription allows the listener to follow what is said, focus on the content, take notes, and review the materials after the session has ended.

Having concrete material to take home helps reinforce the education families receive. Furthermore, these materials can be made available to family members who could not, or would not, attend the education session. It can also be helpful for relatives to look over or review handout materials at home, in an environment that may seem less threatening than the hospital.

Illustrative Educational Presentations

Examples of the four presentations routinely made in the education component of the Brentwood Family Treatment Program have been transcribed and edited and illustrate how approaches studied and applied by others can be adapted to the goals and circumstances of a specific treatment program (see the appendix to this chapter). The content of the topics covered and the general approach used in the presentations derive largely from previous work done by Robert Liberman, Ian Falloon, Gerard Hogarty, Carol Anderson and Sandra Rappé. Dr. Anderson's and Ms. Rappé's work is particularly evident in the section on family and social factors. Our presentations thus reflect the integration of a number of different perspectives, including our own. The program we have developed is only one of many ways in which family education can be developed as an intrinsic component of a family-oriented treatment unit.

References

1. Brown GW, Monck EM, Carstairs GM, et al: Influence of family life on the course of schizophrenic illness. British Journal of Preventive and Social Medicine 16:55–68, 1962

2. Vaughn CE, Leff JP: The influence of family and social factors on the course of psychiatric illness: a comparison of schizophrenic and depressed neurotic patients. Br J Psychiatry 129:125–137, 1976

3. Berkowitz R, Eberlein-Fries R, Kuipers L, et al: Educating relatives about schizophrenia. Schizophr Bull 10:418–429, 1984

4. Berkowitz R, Kuipers L, Eberlein-Fries R, et al: Lowering expressed emotion in relatives of schizophrenics, in New Developments in Interventions with Families of Schizophrenics. Edited by Goldstein MJ. San Francisco, Jossey-Bass, 1981

5. Snyder K, Liberman R: Family assessment and intervention with schizophrenics at risk for relapse, in New Developments in Interventions with Families of Schizophrenics. Edited by Goldstein MJ. San Francisco, Jossey-Bass, 1981

6. Cozolino LJ, Goldstein MJ, Neuchterlein KH: Family education in the psychosocial treatment of schizophrenia. Presented at NIMH workshop on Preventative Intervention Programs for Family Units with a Mentally Ill Member. La Jolla, CA, 1982

7. Falloon I, Boyd JL, McGill C, et al: Family management training in the community care of schizophrenia, in New Developments in Interventions with Families of Schizophrenics. Edited by Goldstein MJ. San Francisco, Jossey-Bass, 1981

8. Anderson CM, Hogarty G, Reiss DJ: The psychoeducational family treatment of schizophrenics, in New Developments in Interventions with Families of Schizophrenics. Edited by Goldstein MJ. San Francisco, Jossey-Bass, 1981

9. Hatfield AB: Help-seeking behavior in families of schizophrenics. Am J Community Psychol 7:563–569, 1979

10. Hatfield AB: Coping effectiveness in families of the mentally ill: an exploratory study. Journal of Psychiatric Treatment and Evaluation 3:11–19, 1981

APPENDIX: ILLUSTRATIVE EDUCATIONAL PRESENTATIONS

The presentations given below were developed by the professional staff of the Family Treatment Program at the West Los Angeles Veterans Administration Medical Center, Brentwood Division. They include the following: "Introduction to Family Education," by Melvin R. Lansky, M.D., Chief Psychiatrist; "Diagnosis and Symptoms," by Kathryn L. West, Ph.D., Clinical Psychologist; "Biology, Neurophysiology, and Pharmacology," by Barnet Malin, M.D., Psychiatry Resident, and "The Family and Social Factors," by Geneva G. McVey, R.N., C., Head Nurse, and Carol R. Bley, M.S.W., Senior Social Worker.

Introduction to Family Education

Good afternoon. I am Dr. Lansky. I am the staff psychiatrist in charge of Ward 206D, the Family Treatment Program at the Brentwood VA Hospital. I want to introduce you to our education program for families of patients who have been diagnosed as having schizophrenia. The purpose of our education program is to offer you the opportunity to learn about the illness called schizophrenia.

Schizophrenia is a very frightening word to most people. It gives rise to wild fantasies that the patient will be totally helpless or totally out of control, or will be doomed to be in a hospital or unable to function for the rest of his or her life. Such fantasies are very far from the truth. They arise from misinformation and hearsay. However, it's easy to see why people are frightened when they are told that their relative has schizophrenia. They don't know what the illness really is, they don't know how it can be expected to affect them, they don't know what can be done about it, and they don't know what the patient can be expected to do or be responsible for. In our education program we will explain about the illness, describe its symptoms, tell you about the course that it takes, and help you see what it is that you, the family, can do to aid in the recovery period after hospitalization.

It is important for you to know that in our opinion families or people in families *do not cause* schizophrenia. We do not know what *does* cause this disorder. We can observe that schizophrenia occurs in some families more often than it does in others, but there are still only a small number of family members related to a schizophrenic who will ever have schizophrenia themselves. There's no reason to think that the illness is related to how one is raised or even to the special kinds of stresses that a person experiences while growing up. In our education program we will be discussing all these matters in more detail.

While we know that families don't cause this illness, we also know that they can help a great deal in keeping the patient out of the hospital after discharge. In addition to providing you with information about the illness, our treatment program is designed to help you understand what it is that you can do to help. Families need to decide what changes they and the patient must make in order for the patient to return to the home after being discharged. Sometimes other steps must be taken first, such as having the patient spend a period of time in a halfway house or a board and care home. There is no one way that is appropriate for all patients and their families. We want to work out with you what will be best for you, so that you don't face an unreasonable regimen that will exhaust all of your resources of time, money, and emotional energy. And, we want to help plan something that will be realistic for your sick relative, so that he or she will be able to live in as satisfying a way as is possible.

Since family education is only one part of the Family Treatment Program, I'd like to describe that program as a whole and what it offers. The ward staff is made up of individuals from various professions, all of whom are an integral part of the treatment team and participate in the treatment decisions. All of them are experienced in working with hospitalized schizophrenic patients, who sometimes need care around the clock. And all of them support the treatment program's focus of working with the patient's families, who can provide us with important input that can help in the patient's treatment.

The psychiatrists on the staff are medical doctors who have special training in psychiatric and emotional illnesses. Their expertise includes the use of medications and the assessment of physical conditions in addition to psychiatric treatment planning, psychotherapy, and, at times, family therapy.

The psychiatric social workers have special skills in dealing with agencies and institutions, and in helping patients find accommodations and jobs and obtain benefits to which they are entitled. In addition, the social workers on Ward 206D are expert psychotherapists with both individuals and families. They often coordinate and supervise, as well as participate in the entire treatment effort being carried out with individual patients and their families.

The clinical psychologists have special expertise in the assessment of psychological and neuropsychological disorders. They, too, provide psychotherapy for individual patients and families and for groups of patients and families. Their skills also include the use of specialized psychological treatments such as relaxation therapy and biofeedback.

The registered psychiatric nurses have special training in administering medications and providing the care that patients need when they are unable to care for themselves. It is the nursing staff that has the most extensive ongoing contact with patients and who provide the moment-by-moment supervision and interactions that patients find so important in helping them recover. Nurses are also trained in individual, group, family, and multiple family therapy.

Ward 206D is organized into three teams, so that each of our three doctors is responsible for only six or seven patients at any one time. Each team includes persons from the different professions who contribute their special skills to the individual patient's treatment. Having a staff team that works together with one small group of patients allows for individualized care and creates cohesive groups in which patients and staff can get to know one another well. In addition, each patient is assigned to a member of the nursing staff, and it is this person to whom the patient can turn whenever it is necessary.

Family members can participate in the treatment program in a number of ways. They are always encouraged to come to the team intake meetings, where, right from the start, they can contribute their knowledge about what has happened to the patient. This information is important for the treatment team to have. For example, family members may have different points of view about the illness, about what brought it on, about what can be accomplished by having the patient hospitalized, or about what will need to be done after the period of hospitalization is over. When there is disagreement within the family or between the family and the patient about such matters, staff can schedule further meetings in which the different views can be better understood and the conflicts resolved. Among the matters that can be decided at team intake meetings is whether or not the patient and family will find it profitable to meet regularly in family therapy sessions.

Families can also participate in multiple family therapy, where groups of families meet together. In such a setting a family can learn a great deal about the difficulties it faces by hearing from other families who have had similar experiences. Families provide each other with useful advice as well as emotional support and empathy.

There may be occasions when the staff will call a special meeting with a family to deal with some unusual circumstance or emergency. Similarly, a family may request a special meeting to consult with staff over new issues that have arisen in the home. Sometimes a family member may want individual counseling, and staff often is able to provide them with this special help.

I hope that this overview of the Family Treatment Program has been helpful and that the family education program which follows will help you to understand more about the baffling, upsetting illness of schizophrenia.

Diagnosis and Symptoms

Good afternoon. My name is Dr. West, and I am the clinical psychologist on the Family Treatment Program. What I want to do is to talk with you about your son's or daughter's illness and help you understand more about it. You may not know this, but 10 percent of the people in this country suffer from some sort of mental illness at some time in their lives. In fact, 50 percent (one-half) of all the people in hospitals in the United States are there because of mental illness. Yet, even though mental illnesses are not uncommon, most people know very little about them.

The illness your son or daughter has is called schizophrenia. Some people think that schizophrenia means a split personality, but that's not what it is at all. A split personality is a symptom of an entirely different mental illness. Schizophrenia is an abnormal condition of the mind. It affects the way you think, the way you feel, and the way you deal with the world, and the result is that people with schizophrenia have a hard time knowing what's real and what's not real.

Schizophrenia shows itself through four different types of typical symptoms. Some patients may have only one type of symptom; others may have two, three, or all four. We want you to understand what these symptoms are so that you'll be better able to understand your son's or daughter's experience of the illness.

First, there are hallucinations. People perceive things, usually voices, when nobody is talking to them. When you have verbal hallucinations, you hear someone talking to you or about you. Sometimes the patient will appear to be talking to himself; what is really happening is that he is carrying on a conversation with a voice that is an hallucination. These are called auditory hallucinations because they involve hearing. There are other kinds of hallucinations, however: seeing things that aren't really there, or feeling or smelling something that isn't really there. These also occur, but hearing voices is the most common hallucination. Imagine how distressing it must be not to know whether what one is experiencing is real or unreal.

Second, there are delusions. A delusion is a belief that seems very real to you but isn't logical or sensible to anyone else. For example, you may be convinced that some other person or force is controlling your actions or thoughts, or you may feel that some other person or thing is out to harm or kill you. Most delusions have this frightening quality to them. If a patient feels under attack or desperately frightened, he or she might strike out or be violent. What appears to us as irrational aggression may be, for the patient, an act of self-protection. Of course, we must always remember that not every notion or belief that a schizophrenic patient has is necessarily delusional. Sometimes patients are taken advantage of, just as other persons are. The problem lies in helping them know what is real and what is the result of their illness.

The third kind of symptom is called "thought disorder." This refers to the wide variety of experiences that patients have which can result in strange ways of communicating and behaving. These thoughts and actions indicate that the way someone with schizophrenia perceives and experiences the world about him and what happens to him when he tries to communicate with other people are different from what people usually experience.

A frequently experienced thought disorder is having a problem with attention. Most of us can concentrate on something fairly well if we really want to, and even when we're distracted we can get back to what we were doing without too much trouble. A person with schizophrenia finds this far more difficult. Something that would be trivial to us is a major distraction for him. Here's how patients have described what happens:[1]

> "If something else is going on somewhere, even just a noise, it interrupts my thoughts and they get lost." "If I'm talking to someone and they just cross their legs or scratch their head, I'm distracted and forget what I was saying."

When a patient is trying to think about something or follow a conversation, this is what can happen:

> "I can concentrate if they talk simple. When they go into long sentences, I lose the meanings." "My thoughts wander off or get stuck or seem all jumbled up."

Another mental process that is the result of the psychosis is the distortion of sights and sounds. For example:

> "Noises all seem to be louder to me than they were before. It's as if someone had turned up the volume." "I'm not sure if things are solid until I touch them." "Colors seem clearer, yet at the same time something is missing."

The psychotic process can also affect the patient's experience of his body and its movement. They've described it this way:

> "If there's too much noise going on, I can't move. It's almost as if I am paralyzed." "When I move quickly or unexpectedly, it stuns me, like a shock." "If I move fast, I feel like everything would break up and be a jumbled mass." "I'm not sure of my own movements any more, even simple actions like sitting down. This makes me move much slower now."

---

[1] The quotations produced here are either verbatim or adapted from patients' descriptions published in McGhie A, Chapman J: Disorders of attention and perception in early schizophrenia. Br J Med Psychol 34:103–116, 1961.

You can imagine how emotionally disturbing these experiences are for the patient. They cause severe depression. They are also frightening, and when symptoms of thought disorder are present, a patient may threaten other people or even strike out, because he feels himself to be in danger. This is something that is particularly troubling to families—not knowing if the patient will lose control and be a danger to himself or to others.

A fourth set of symptoms is what we call social isolation. By this we mean a pattern of behaviors that are not sociable and that may be socially unacceptable. Many schizophrenic patients tend to stay alone, to retreat into a private world, to find it hard to talk or even to be with other people, including members of the family. It's also hard for most schizophrenics to find any interest in work or in going to school; they simply don't have the drive or motivation to get involved or make what, for them, is an enormous effort. To other people, they seem lazy, but their isolation and inability to become involved is not laziness. It's a symptom of their illness. It is not unusual, either, for a person with schizophrenia to have no interest even in keeping himself clean or well-groomed. Nor is it unusual for him to behave in public in ways that are considered uncouth or disgusting by most people. Such behaviors are difficult for families and friends to understand, let alone accept, but they are common symptoms of schizophrenia. It's as though nothing can really matter to the patient except the strange and often terrifying things that are going on inside his or her head.

I think you can imagine how difficult it would be if you had any or all of these symptoms. How could you live a normal life that involved concentrating on work, studying diligently, or socializing easily with friends, when it was impossible for you to keep your mind on a task, to plan ahead, to ignore the hallucinations and delusions you are experiencing, and to keep from feeling completely out of control?

Fortunately, some of the symptoms I've described can be relieved with drugs. Dr. Malin, who will talk with you next, will discuss how drugs and medications fit into the treatment of schizophrenia. Unfortunately, there is little that medications can do to help the fourth set of symptoms I've just described: the social isolation, the withdrawal, the absence of drive or ambition, and the lack of caring about one's appearance or habits. What is needed for these problems is other kinds of treatment, and this is where the family can be of enormous help. Recently there have been some excellent research studies that have demonstrated just how helpful the family can be. People with schizophrenia are easily upset by emotional turmoil and stress. When upsetting things occur, their symptoms get worse and they have to be hospitalized. When stress can be kept down, it's possible for them to live and function outside the hospital. Our goal, then, is to help them avoid the situations that are stressful for them, and we can go far toward accomplishing this goal when families are willing to work along with us.

One of the first things we have to do is to help the patient and the family figure out what is stressful and what is not, what he can do for himself and what he can't realistically be expected to do, since these issues may be different in every case. By meeting together, the patient, the family, and the staff can work out how to make things better. After you've heard from Dr. Malin, Mrs. McVey and Ms. Bley will speak with you in more detail about the ways in which we work with families on this treatment unit.

I want to close with a bit of history—both ancient and modern. Schizophrenia has been around for centuries, and people in all periods of history have struggled to understand it and deal with persons suffering from it. Hundreds of years ago they thought that it was caused by witches or the devil. In the early 1900s, some doctors believed that it was caused by rotten teeth, so a fair number of schizophrenics had their teeth extracted—to no avail, I should add. More recently, people have thought that schizophrenia was caused by social or psychological factors, such as the way a child was raised by his parents. These theories all have one thing in common: we don't believe any of them. Schizophrenia isn't caused by families, by the devil, by witches, or by rotten teeth!

What remains troublesome, however, is that even today there are treatments being offered that haven't proven to be any better than pulling teeth. And because families are so desperate to find what they hope will be a cure for the illness, some will try anything. One treatment currently being offered is megavitamin therapy, based on the idea that large doses of vitamins will cure schizophrenia. Another is called renal dialysis, a procedure for artificially purifying the blood. This is a legitimate procedure used in some kidney diseases, but it's not a treatment for schizophrenia. Another popular treatment is called "rebirthing." It's based on the notion that a person can be "talked" into returning to the time of his actual birth so that he can relive his life, this time without a mental illness. We don't believe that these or some other currently popular treatments for schizophrenia are effective. However, you deserve to know that they exist and what our views of them are, because you are almost certain to hear of them.

Biology, Neurophysiology, and Pharmacology

Good afternoon. My name is Dr. Malin, and I am a psychiatrist on the Family Treatment Program. I'd like to speak with you today about the biological, or physical, aspects of schizophrenia. We've come a long way in our understanding of some of the problems in the brain and nervous system that occur in schizophrenia, and will present to you some important points concerning both biological problems and use of medications. However, we are really just beginning to understand these topics, and it is important for all of you to realize the limitations of our knowledge. In fact, these limitations are one of the main reasons that family involvement in the treatment of schizophrenia is so helpful.

To sum up the most important point: the management of medications is best accomplished as a collaboration between patient, doctor, and family. In our education program today, we hope to make this collaboration understandable and easier to do.

To start off, let's take a look at the diagram I've handed out to you (Figure 1). Here you see drawings of two pairs of cells in the brain, called "neurons." The brain has billions of cells in it, and there are many more in the spinal cord and the rest of the neurologic system. One function of the neurologic system is to transmit information to and from all points in the body. This is important to know, because our understanding of what goes wrong in the brain in schizophrenia has to do with faulty transmission of information from one cell, or neuron, to another.

How does information get transferred from one neuron to another? In the diagram you have, look at the space between the cells. This space is called a synapse. The way that messages are sent from one cell to another is through a little package of chemicals that goes across the space from the first neuron to the second neuron. Here's what happens: a small electric charge is sent down the arm of the first neuron, right to the end of the cell. This causes a package of chemicals to be released into the synapse. You can think of this in a couple of ways. For example, think of a baseball pitcher who winds up to deliver the pitch; that's like the electric charge reaching the end of the cell. The ball then flies through the air; that's like the package of chemicals crossing the synapse. Then the ball goes right to the catcher's mitt; that's like the package of chemicals fitting into the receptor on the second neuron.

There's a second way to think about it, also. Instead of using pitchers, baseballs, and catchers, think about spaceships. Let's say there is a space capsule and a space station with a docking port. In order to link up, the capsule must go into the docking port. It can't dock in the space station's window or door. Also, it must be lined up perfectly with the docking port so that it will fit properly. The same idea applies to the chemical package and the receptor on the neuron. Each package fits with a special receptor, built and shaped especially for it, and when it fits in the right way, the electric signal begins its journey down the second cell. When the charge reaches the end of the cell, the whole process starts again. This is how neurons communicate with each other, both in people who have schizophrenia and in those who do not.

Now we need to consider what it is that goes wrong in schizophrenia. The name of the chemical in the package we are interested in is dopamine. The problem, as best as we understand it, is that too much information gets transmitted through the dopa-

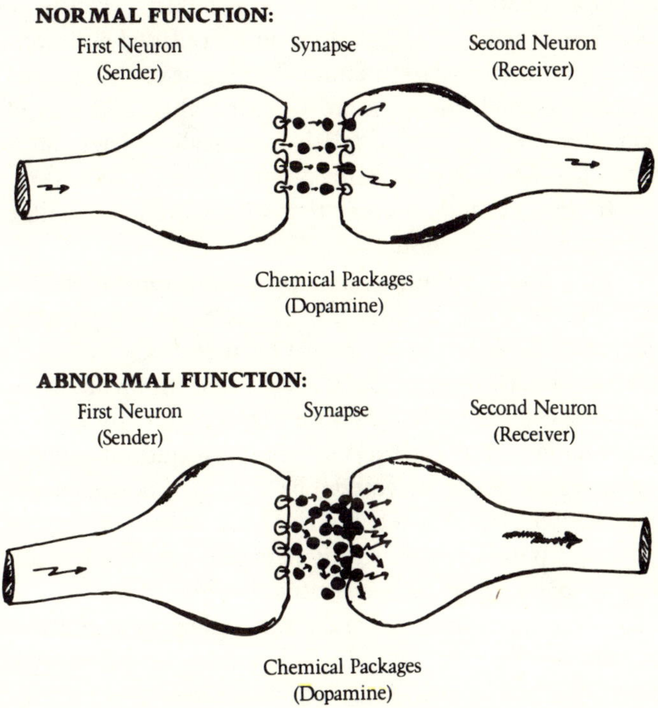

Figure 1. Diagram of two neurons.

mine system. This could be because there is too much dopamine around. It might mean that there are too many dopamine receptors around. Or, it might mean that each dopamine package and receptor transmits more information than usual.

Whatever the reason, the result is that there is just too much information to handle. It's like watching five movies at once, or being on a party line where everyone is talking. For the person involved, this overload of information is confused and nonsensical. At times it may be frightening. The name of this condition is "psychosis," which means a break with reality, and a psychotic person is one who is out of touch with reality. There are other psychiatric illnesses besides schizophrenia in which people may be psychotic, but you should know that schizophrenia is an illness in which people are psychotic.

Knowing about dopamine and how communication is transmitted gives us a way of understanding some of the symptoms of schizophrenia. We call these "positive symptoms." "Positive" does not mean "good," in this case; it means that things are there that normally shouldn't be. For instance, it is common for people with schizophrenia to hear voices. With an excess amount of dopamine communication going on, could it be that the abnormal dopamine messages might be interpreted in the brain as an actual voice? We don't know if this is the way it happens, but this formulation seems to make sense. Other positive symptoms include disconnected or confused thoughts and bizarre attempts at communication such as saying strange things or making up words. Another positive symptom is delusions, which are ideas and feelings that people have that are true to them but not true to others. For instance, someone may be convinced that the FBI has sent agents to follow him. Still another positive symptom is violent and assaultive behavior. (There are still other symptoms which are called "negative symptoms," and I will mention them later.)

We can now understand the function of medications in the treatment of schizophrenia. There are several names that describe the medications used. Probably the best name is "antipsychotic," for it accurately describes what the medication does—it works to decrease psychosis. Other names include "neuroleptics" and "phenothiazines." An old name, which is sometimes still used but is inappropriate, is "major tranquilizer." As you now know, the primary action of these medications is not tranquilization or sedation but the reduction of psychosis.

We believe that the medications work by reducing the amount of dopamine-mediated information in the brain. It appears that the medications fit into the dopamine receptor and keep the dopamine from getting in. This prevents the communication of dopamine-mediated information, and, we think, decreases the overload of psychotic information that the untreated schizophrenic person receives. This decrease in mental stimulation allows the schizophrenic person to filter out irrelevant, confusing signals, which lets them concentrate more effectively and be in touch with reality.

There are many kinds of neuroleptics, but they all work in the way I've just described. Some of the names you may have heard are Thorazine, Haldol, Mellaril, Prolixin, Navane, Loxitane, Stelazine, Trilafon. These are all brand names, just as "Kleenex" is a brand name for facial tissue. You may also have heard a few of the chemical names, like chlorpromazine or haloperidol. The very first neuroleptic, chlorpromazine, which was marketed by the name Thorazine, was developed in the 1950s and found to have great usefulness, and we still use Thorazine today. These medications changed the treatment of schizophrenia forever. Most people are now treated in an outpatient setting instead of living their lives in hospitals.

All of the medications are equally effective. They differ, however, in how potent they are. You can think of potency as a measure of how concentrated the medication is. It takes more of a low-potency, or weakly concentrated medication, to get the same effect as a smaller amount of a high-potency, or highly concentrated medication. For instance, it might take 10 mg of a high-potency medication to get exactly the same effect as 500 mg of a low-potency medication. Common high-potency medications include Haldol, Prolixin, and Navane. Common low-potency medications are Thorazine and Mellaril. Medications like Stelazine, Trilafon, and Loxitane fall in between.

How do we choose one medication over another? There are several factors to be considered, including the physician's experience with the different drugs. There are also special cases. For example, Prolixin comes in a form which can be given as a shot once every one or two weeks. That makes this medication good for people who, for whatever reasons, can't take pills every day.

A major reason for choosing one medication rather than another for any individual patient is the different side effects of the drugs. It is important to understand that almost any kind of medication may have side effects. A common drug like aspirin may cause bleeding or even death from an allergic reaction, but side effects from aspirin are extremely rare, and aspirin is still sold in supermarkets. Most of the side effects of the antipsychotics are not dangerous. However, they are very uncomfortable and, unfortunately, they are common. It is not possible to predict how sensitive any individual person may be to particular side effects. This is one of the most important reasons for an educational program such as this. As I said earlier, the use of medication for people with schizophrenia must be a collaborative effort between patient, doctor, and, if possible, the family. In this way the proper dose, meaning not too much and not too little, may be achieved with a minimum number of uncomfortable side effects or, as is often possible, no side effects at all.

The high-potency medications tend to have several common side effects. One is what is called the "restless leg" syndrome, or "akithisia." This is an uncomfortable urge to move around, or an inability to find a comfortable position. The person's restlessness may look like anxiety to others but, in fact, may be this side effect. A second side effect is just the opposite, called the "stiffness syndrome," in which a person seems rigid. They may sit extremely still, without the little movements we usually make, and they may walk with stiff arms or a stiff gait. We treat both of these side effects by giving another medication along with the antipsychotics. The medications we use include Cogentin, Artane, Akineton, Symmetrel, and Benadryl.

The low-potency medications differ from the high-potency medications in that sedation tends to be more common than the restless leg or stiffness syndromes. This might make low-potency medications preferable for someone who is always agitated or sleepless.

There can also be side effects such as dry mouth, light-headedness when arising, reversible impotence, and weight gain. Weight gain seems to occur with most medications, though not with every person. If someone experiences impotence, he should tell his doctor, and a medication change can be made. It is also important to let the doctor know if someone is light-headed, since that might mean that the person's blood pressure is too low.

An uncommon reaction from the high-potency medications is called a "dystonic reaction," which means that right after a dose, a person may have muscle spasms in the neck muscles or eye muscles, or sometimes the body. This is easily treated with an injection.

There is one serious long-term side effect you must know about. It is called "tardive dyskinesia." Tardive dyskinesia is most often caused by excessive doses of antipsychotic medications taken over a long period of time, usually years. Sometimes, though, it can occur with small doses of medications over short periods of time. The side effect starts with abnormal movements, smacking movements of the lips and tongue, and many times this is all that happens. If it progresses, however, abnormal movements of the hands or body may occur. Since these changes can become permanent, doctors usually decrease the amount of the medication. Currently there are many research studies underway looking for a treatment for this side effect. Meanwhile, the prevention and early detection of tardive dyskinesia is extremely important and is another reason that close collaboration is essential in the medication treatment of schizophrenia.

I want to mention, also, a few other areas that people always have questions about. One is the use and effects of street drugs and alcohol. The use of street drugs is dangerous for people with schizophrenia, for the drug may cause a worsening of symptoms, especially disorganized thinking. When a person is acutely psychotic, all street drugs are harmful in that they confuse the person even more and may lead to dangerous behavior. As for alcohol, people who take antipsychotic medication are particularly susceptible to its effects, and it is easier for them to become drunk.

In talking about medications I've described their usefulness in reducing the positive symptoms of schizophrenia that occur during its acute phase. When people with schizophrenia receive treatment and are in remission, the positive symptoms are greatly diminished and may even disappear completely. What is important for you to know is that medications are effective in keeping the florid symptoms of the illness away. They can help prevent the positive symptoms from coming back and keep people from getting acutely sick again. This is important to know, because many people understandably want to stop taking their medications once they feel okay. They say, "I'm not sick now, so I don't need the medications." Unfortunately, the relapse rate is much higher when people do not continue taking their medications. Without medication, the transmission problems in the synapse, which I described earlier, will return.

Helpful as medications are, unfortunately they cannot make the illness go away, and sometimes people can get psychotic again, even while they are on medications. This may necessitate a hospitalization to reevaluate the dose and choice of medication.

Earlier I mentioned that there are negative symptoms in schizophrenia in addition to the positive ones that are helped by medications. Dr. West has already described them in some detail—the withdrawal, the isolation, the low or absent motivation to do things, and so forth. Let me remind you that medications do not seem to help these symptoms as much as they help the positive ones. It is other therapies, such as family therapy, living skills training, and certain types of counseling that are needed for dealing with the negative symptoms.

I hope that this talk has been informative and interesting. With this brief introduction you now have been exposed to the most important biological and medical facts about the illness of schizophrenia. I would be glad to answer any questions you may have. Thank you for listening.

The Family and Social Factors

Hello. We are Geneva McVey and Carol Bley, Head Nurse and Senior Social Worker on the Family Treatment Program. Our topic is schizophrenia and the family. To emphasize what others have already said, there is no evidence that families cause this illness, but there is good evidence that a family can do many things that will help the patient during the recovery process.

We will take turns sharing some of our observations with you and making some recommendations to you. We hope our suggestions will be helpful, but we also know that you will learn a great deal by sharing your experiences with one another. Keep in mind that if you have any problems, please call us. Our staff is available 24 hours a day to assist you with suggestions or advice.

Living with the patient. Most of you have had the experience of being with your relative during the acute phase of the illness, a time when your relative was hearing voices, seeing unreal things, expressing strange thoughts, and being extremely frightened or upset. During such times, difficult as they may be, it is not hard to be sympathetic with your relative because it is obvious that the person is suffering from the acute phase of a psychiatric illness. Knowing this sometimes makes it easier for you to accept the situation and deal with it.

However, after the acute phase of the illness has passed and the patients are no longer plagued by hallucinations, delusions, and thought disturbances, it can become difficult for their families to understand why they do not now act as they did before. One can't help wondering: Why is the patient unable to work or at least share in the chores around the house? Why is the patient so withdrawn and unsociable? Why is the patient so neglectful of personal appearance and hygiene when looking neat and clean mattered so much before? Since the patient now is no longer *acutely* ill, relatives have difficulty remembering that the patient has a *chronic* illness and is *still* sick.

Things to remember. Your relatives are not well, even though they may appear to be okay. They have been and still are seriously ill, and it will take quite a while before they are able to do many of the things they once handled easily. They may now spend more time alone in their rooms than they used to. They may talk with you less often. They may pace. They may be restless and move around constantly. They may suddenly get up and leave the dining room table during dinner. These behaviors will be different from what you are accustomed to, but they are very much a part of the illness.

Changing expectations. The fact that your sons or daughters have a psychotic illness makes it necessary for you to change your expectations of what they can do, now and in the future. Perhaps your relative will never be able to obtain that master's degree that was planned or follow the career that was once hoped for. This is bound to be disappointing for you, as it is for the patient. What's important to remember is that the patients and you must change your expectations and find more realistic goals. It will take time to discover what each individual patient can be expected to accomplish. They need to take on responsibilities gradually rather than try to do what they did before. Supporting them as they increase their activities step by step will help build their skills and self-confidence. It's difficult to predict what may be too difficult or too stressful for a patient, so we hope you'll let us help you. Knowing each patient as we do, we may be able to help you and the patient define appropriate short-term and long-term goals for the patient.

Striking a balance. Work toward a balance between what you expect of the patients and what they are able and/or willing to do. Listen to what they tell you. For example, if they say that they are unable to help with work around the house, do not force the issue. Instead, ask them what they feel they can do and let them do just that. They may not be able to complete their chores as well as you would like, but they deserve your appreciation for whatever it is they are able to accomplish.

Keep the level of emotion down. When at all possible, avoid emotional scenes, which are always stressful for patients. Try not to argue with them, especially about their experiences. Their strange ideas and feelings, their irrational thoughts and fears—these are symptoms of the illness. Suppose your relative tries to convince you that you can see something that isn't there. Express your view and let it go at that. Simply say, "I know that you think you see something, but I don't." Remember that conflict is stressful. It can make their symptoms worse and can even bring them on.

Keep things simple and predictable. Patients find it difficult to handle complexities and unexpected change, so keep things as simple and predictable as possible. When you speak, be brief and clear so that your messages are easy to understand. Try to do things on a regular schedule, for this allows the patient to cope more easily with the routines around the home. Try to be predictable in what you do, yourself. If you make promises, keep them.

Be firm but gentle about medication and appointments. You can be helpful to the patients if you monitor their medication schedules and hospital appointments, but that doesn't mean you need to take all the responsibility for them. Find ways to remind the patient without being a nag. Some families have found it helpful to have a medication chart or appointment schedule posted in some convenient place, like on the refrigerator door. It's helpful to keep the medication in a readily visible and available place where just seeing it can serve as a reminder to the patient. If it is still necessary for you to remind the patient frequently, do so without being critical.

Encourage what can be done. There are many simple things that patients can do for themselves, but they need your encouragement and praise for doing so and your compliments when they make even small improvements in how they manage a task. Don't expect them to do things perfectly. For example, let them make their beds in their own way; if the corners aren't folded properly or the pillow isn't in the right place, let it go! Tell them you're pleased at what they have done, and leave it at that.

Go on with your own life. It is important for you to continue doing the things that bring you pleasure and satisfaction. Your relative faces a long recovery period, and no one expects you to give up things that are important to you during this time. Visit friends, go shopping, take classes, work on your hobbies, keep up whatever activities you enjoy doing. You will be of more help to your relative if you take care of yourself, keep up your own health, and pursue your own pleasures.

Family support groups. It is our experience that families can gain a great deal of help and information from support groups like the multiple family group on our unit or others that are available in the community. These groups are made up of families with a mentally ill relative. They have a great deal to offer. Families who share difficulties and concerns can often provide each other with more help and comfort than they can get from other relatives or friends, or even from us professionals! We have information about support groups for you and will provide you with this at the end of the meeting.

Let us help. Every family who has a mentally ill relative has problems, and we want to do whatever we can to help. Please contact us whenever you have questions or need to discuss problems that arise. Thank you for coming.

5

Family Psychotherapy of the Patient with Chronic Organic Brain Syndrome

Melvin R. Lansky, M.D.

5

Family Psychotherapy of the Patient with Chronic Organic Brain Syndrome

TREATMENT ISSUES

Dementia is usually assumed by the the therapist to be an irreversible organic brain syndrome (OBS). This assumption typifies the premature closure that is prevalent in the treatment of OBS patients. Often the brain dysfunction is compounded by old age, somatic problems, a family situation in which the patient is helpless and anxious, and depression from many sources including awareness of self as lacking in cognitive faculties. Such a predicament often seems to the therapist something that can be responded to only with support rather than with definitive psychotherapy. It seems psychostatic rather than psychodynamic. The pathology is irreversible. A deficit due to brain disease may not reverse or improve and may seem to have no relationship to interpersonal activities. By and large such patients are uninteresting to therapists because their future possibilities seem so small. The fact that the deficit is in the mind itself makes both therapist's and patient's responses different from those elicited by other chronic illnesses. The patient's mental capacity, the very target of

Reprinted from Psychiatric Annals 14:121–129, 1984, with the kind permission of SLACK Inc. and Dr. Norman Q. Brill.

interpretive work and understanding, is itself permanently damaged.

However, behind these issues suggestive of a static situation often lurk more deeply seated ones that impede seeing intervention as helpful to the overall picture (1). The therapist, for one reason or another, may confuse the difficulties facing the patient or the family with the actual cerebral pathology, and overlook or withdraw from interventions that decisively change the overall morbidity caused by the disorder. This avoidance on the therapist's part may be due to a simple inability to assess the situation from the point of view of the family, or from basic discomfort in working with families or other systems. Discomfort with family systems may accompany similar difficulties with other systems important in the patient's life, such as hospitals, other institutions, extended family, and other helping persons, that may be understood within a systems framework.

Any lack of skill as a disciplined psychotherapist, especially in tolerating and working with severe countertransference reactions, may further impede the therapist's ability to view the therapeutic work as productive or even decisive. The therapist may be overwhelmed, feel futile, and withdraw too soon. Countertransference factors include the therapist's guilt at having an intact mental apparatus when he or she is face to face with a patient who is deteriorating.

It may be difficult to get close to a patient whose progress is not gratifying and who may be depressed or unable to converse well. Therapists may be swept up in feelings of helplessness or in the panic generated by the family of the patient with organic brain disease, because they feel too many demands, or too much guilt about caring for such a patient. The therapist should be able to identify and modify fantasies about what is involved in the care of such a person; frequently the patient's needs are felt in fantasy to be inexhaustible and the patient is seen as someone requiring endless care, never improving, using up resources, limiting other people's possibilities, and enduring for many years as a constant drain. In the face of all of these, the therapist may overreact to feelings of futility, resentment, panic, and a misguided notion of what is required in the care of such patients.[1] By being overreactive, the therapist runs the risk of becoming overwhelmed, feeling repulsed and futile, and abandoning the therapeutic scene too soon and with an incomplete view of the situation. The danger is particularly great because overreaction in those cases usually consists of giving up; the therapist can rationalize this futility as appropriate to the cerebral pathology itself and does not see himself or herself as being reactive.

The situation is, of course, more complex if the therapist is wrestling with unresolved issues—often with his or her own parents: their decline, their demands, feelings of guilt about superseding parents or about not doing enough for them. These lead to mis-estimates of what is actually required and pessimism about any amelioration at all. If these issues are unresolved, the therapist is often unable to help the family because he lacks the ability to model and vocalize what the family cannot say, and is unable to face fantasies about the greediness of heirs, the wish for death of the patient and consequent guilt, and wishes about release from caretaking, to name some of the fantasies that commonly arise in the family.

The treatment of the patient with dementia is almost never the province of a psychotherapist alone. There are usually medical illnesses to contend with. There are institutions and social systems including agencies, hospitals, lawyers, extended family members, nursing homes, all of which may exert pressure on the family system, and in turn on the patient. Both family members and institutions fear being blamed, fear having demands made on them, and vie for a favorable position in terms of their own family or institutional system. Not only must individual and family therapy be considered but also interventions requiring comprehension of the entire systems or networks of systems of which the

---

[1] A striking picture of the overwhelmed reaction of caretakers to OBS patients is to be found in Samuel Shem's *The House of God* (2). The novel portrays an internship year and deals unabashedly with the intern's severe emotional reaction to "gomers"—aged patients who are uncommunicative, needy, demented, and in need of care, and who neither die nor improve, but present insatiable demands for caretaking.

patient is a part. In this network the psychotherapist may be felt to be of low rank, either a nonmedical person, or a medical person assumed to be auxiliary in the bigger picture. Extraordinary pressure may be placed on the therapist to deal with larger systems in which he or she is not in control.

The field of dyadic individual psychotherapy may be too limited to be effective. The pathology itself brings forth defenses such as denial and confabulation that protect against catastrophic reactions (3) and shame (4). These, coupled with the cognitive deficits themselves, may disorganize efforts at individual therapy. The therapist treating such a patient in isolation is likely to feel demands of the situation heavily and either overregulate the patient or become exhausted and withdraw from the treatment or confine it to simply reassuring endeavors. The project of freeing the patient up from repetitive and unproductive parts of interpersonal process becomes a very murky concept unless it is seen from the perspective of the entire family system.

For these reasons family-focused treatment must be considered the treatment of choice for the patient with dementia. The family provides the best setting to see what containment functions have to be exercised by the family when the patient's usual personality functions or cognitive functions have declined. By examining what the family does, feels it has to do, and realistically has to do, the therapist is in a better position to see the impact of the family process on the patient, and the impact of the patient on family process. These are often off-handedly assumed to be irrelevant in the treatment of the patient with organic brain disease, but close examination will reveal that they are important in the vast majority of families of OBS patients. Irrational responses, or responses not dictated by the cerebral pathology alone, abound. The therapist can reduce the overall morbidity—for the patient as well as those around him—by helping to clarify some of these issues. Often the patient's condition can be made worse by things that the family does, and it is no rarity to have family members behave in such a way as to agitate a patient whom they can no longer tolerate into actually requiring some custodial situation, even though the cerebral pathology itself does not strictly necessitate such care. If the therapist is swept up in the escalation of symptomatology and accepts an explanation that the panic and helplessness are due to cerebral disorder alone, he or she is likely to overlook the interpersonal processes and succumb to irrational action rather than a realistic estimate of what is required and by whom.

The family also provides a basis for comparison with other systems that support the patient, and the therapist can get an advantageous view of other emotional fields by inquiring what family members think is required of them as caretakers. This may be compared with other caretaking systems—for example, hospitals and nursing homes. Both similarities and differences are noteworthy. A similar response by several different systems points to the patient's role in the difficulties. A different response—for example, if the patient is cooperative on a hospital ward but agitated at home—invites investigation of what in the family system accounts for the difference (see Case Example 3 below).

The therapist of the OBS patient has to face many issues within the family that may be addressed psychotherapeutically and definitively worked through. The following is a partial list:

Ignorance About the Illness

Family ignorance about the illness often extends to not knowing whether it is progressive, whether the patient will require extended care, and so forth—that is, they are sometimes ignorant of the nature and course, and even genetics, of the illness. The family of an OBS patient is frequently not informed about diagnoses and prognoses, often because such patients get insufficient work-up to distinguish cortical from subcortical disease processes. In the absence of a complete work-up, deterioration may be referred to as "aging" or "senility" rather than in terms of a specific diagnosis that carried with it prognosis and treatment response. There may also be ignorance about responsibility: what the patient can do, and for what he can be held responsible. Frequently fantasies abound within the family that the patient can be responsible for absolutely nothing and should be cared for totally, when indeed the patient is capable of assuming many responsibilities that have not been made explicit or agreed upon. An educational component with patients with dementia, whether or not the etiology is known, should be vigorously pursued with the family early in the treatment. They may anticipate memory loss, incontinence, suspiciousness, and even hitting, and must be told that in severely impaired patients simple activities such as cooking, smoking, and driving may now be dangerous (5).

Denial

Often the patient's deeply rooted defense mechanisms against awareness of organic brain deficit are buttressed by the family's reluctance to discuss the deficits in a tactful way that does not unnecessarily humiliate the patient. The family may be needed to minimize the effects of the patient's denial. They should be consulted about whether the patient can go shopping, find his way home, balance a checkbook, be left alone, care for himself, remain continent, and so forth. Often the patient's catastrophic reactions, rage, and confabulations are not addressed by the family. Such problems may be compounded by any difficulties in communication that existed before the cerebral pathology.

Irrational Role Assignments

Often, a family homeostasis involves rigid role assignments that become debilitating when a significant member of the family has an organic brain disease that interferes with enacting such a role.

Case Example 1

A retired colonel was admitted for a work-up that led to a diagnosis of Alzheimer's disease. He had been successful in the military, forceful and decisive in financial matters, and both leader and tyrant at home. His wife was an exceedingly attractive woman two decades his junior, who was accustomed to serving as hostess at many social functions but took no responsibility for the family's financial affairs and made no major decisions. Both rather enjoyed the role assignments, and the marriage was satisfactory to both. However, the decline of the hus-

> band's cognitive capacities left his wife overwhelmed. She could not function, refused to have him discharged from the hospital, attacked the staff, got unnecessary consultations, and bombarded the hospital administrators with complaints. After many family sessions, and finally individual psychotherapy sessions, she could face the shame and depression stemming from her own sense of inadequacy and traceable to her family of origin. This had never been a problem in her marriage before the husband's illness. She had enjoyed her relationship with a dominant and overfunctioning man and had to slowly learn to develop herself in areas that had never before been her responsibility.

Similarly, it is common for daughters of women with OBS to have difficulty in reversing lifelong roles when they find they must mother their mothers.

Failure of Integration in the Family, and Failure of a Sense of Justice

Once the central cohesion formerly provided by a senior family member with organic brain disease is gone, fantasies run rife in the family. Children often worry that others will either get more of the money or property or leave them with the caretaking. Even in cohesive families with much good will, such fantasies are rampant. So are feelings of guilt about fantasied triumph over aged parents and fears that insatiable demands will be made, that people will criticize, that certain family members will be left to care for the patient, and many others. Reactions to aggressive fantasies include guilt, depression, withdrawal when overwhelmed, and inability to talk straightforwardly about what is required of various members in the family.

Retardation of Maturation

Often, organic brain disease in one family member blocks efforts of one or more other family members to separate. Their centrifugal force is inhibited because of what the patient requires, or the patient himself may be unable to separate because of the illness.

Case Example 2

A 37-year-old divorced man had a respiratory arrest with enough cerebral anoxia to cause moderate brain damage. His cardiovascular situation improved, but he had a lasting cerebral deficit. Since his wife and children were no longer in the picture, he was thrown back into a dependent relationship on his parents. The parental marriage was extraordinarily pathological. Although the parents had been divorced for many years, they still lived near each other. The father, a pathologically paranoid man, spent most of his time with the patient's mother, a woman who suffered from a chronic debilitating illness. The father rationalized his difficulty separating by saying that she needed caretaking and noting his guilt about having left her when the patient was eleven. The patient, one of the two children of the marriage, had been the one most drawn in by the marital difficulties. He was left with a good deal of pathological dependency resulting from his involvement in the marriage. After great difficulty, he had separated from his parents in his 20s and married. His own marriage was not successful, and the subsequent cerebral difficulty threw him back into the original family situation, again dependent on his parents. The cerebral deficit was compounded by a serious depression (or pseudodementia) (6), which responded very well to antidepressant medication until his mother took him off the medication and had him admitted to another hospital, where he was placed on a different kind of medication.

The patient himself, a spouse, children, or even parents may be unable to leave or to find gratification away from the family, especially if the family is narcissistically vulnerable or overly enmeshed prior to the illness. In such cases, family members find it hard to extricate themselves from the doings of other people and to have areas of their lives that are separate. When cerebral illness strikes, this enmeshment may become a disaster.

Intensification of Preexisting Family Issues

Often preexisting family issues are compensated or partially worked through but become manifestly pathological after the onset of the illness (Case Examples 1 and 2). Other situations include: intensification of Oedipal rivalry, and especially guilt over the feeling of triumph when a parent declines; overreaction or assumption of complete caretaking roles by one family member, who eventually becomes exhausted, resentful, and angry or depressed in response to the burden (especially if this person has depressive propensities in his personality and cannot negotiate some reasonable adaptation); chronic marital rifts that may decompensate when one member has an organic brain syndrome (7). Marital equilibrium may be kept by constant marital conflict, or impulsive drinking that holds the family together, or by one spouse being constantly absorbed in work functions felt to be valuable for the family. When one person in these collusive transactions becomes demented, the entire defensive system may collapse.

These preexisting difficulties become even worse if there is a lack of negotiating skills in the family. This often happens when the family is naive, overly repressed, or extremely religious in its background, or extremely narcissistically vulnerable and prone to collusive relationships that cannot be discussed.

Blame and Demands

Blame and demands, felt to come from other people but also emanating from self-reproaches, may lead family members to see themselves as required to do endless things for patients, so that eventually they become overwhelmed. Often this sense of blame and demand is projected by the family onto caretakers, especially the hospital, and a situation occurs where the family will put pressure on the patient to be dysfunctional so that the hospital will take over. This is an example of what Murray Bowen has called "triangling," that is, the hospital is felt to balance an unstable relationship between patient and family (8).

Case Example 3

A psychiatric consultant was called to evaluate a 73-year-old man in a hospital after cataract surgery and to arrange for transfer to a psychiatric service or a nursing home because of recurrent psychotic episodes and the ward's fear of violence. The patient had been hospitalized earlier at the family's demand, for the same difficulties. Examination during the day revealed a calm man with mild to moderate brain impairment, but capable of grooming himself and comporting himself reasonably. The psychiatrist met with the ward staff and with the family, and suggested changes: substitution of a neuroleptic for a sedative given at night when the difficulties occurred, keeping lights and radio on, and moving the patient near the nurses' station so that there would be people around. Much improvement was reported the next morning, and the patient was discharged a few days later. However, a few weeks later the patient was readmitted. Despite careful instructions by the psychiatrist, the patient was kept by the family in a dark, lonely part of the house and given sedatives. A psychotic episode ensued, and the patient was returned to the emergency room, where again, he was kept in a dark part of the ward, given sedatives, and had another psychotic episode. The psychiatrist repeated the advice, but eventually the family complained to the hospital director about poor care given to the patient, and the difficulties were compounded.

Misestimation of Patient as Playing Passive Instead of Active Role

Case Example 2 (continued)

The 37-year-old patient put enormous pressure on his parents by running off to the home of a former girlfriend, and running away from the hospital back to his parents' home. This and other activities showed quite clearly that his cognitive deficits, although significant, did not preclude enormous activity on his part to provoke his parents and hospital caretakers and to discharge the hostility he felt about the dependent relationship he had with both.

The patient with organic brain disease may be extraordinarily humiliated at his new dependency and helplessness and may exploit the new situation, enviously attack caretakers, and control those around him who believe him to be passive and incompetent. The patient's shame at his newly dependent predicament cannot be stressed too strongly. Often the patient will not seem to understand that his obtuseness is a method of controlling and discharging hostility that may be mistaken for a cognitive deficit.

Impact of the Process on the Patient

The patient's increased dependency and shame, often compounded by envy and hostility toward caretakers, may result in a depression, the effects of which are superimposed on the cerebral pathology. Such pseudodementia was found in Cases 1 and 2 and responded well to specific treatment for depression—in Case 1, electroconvulsive therapy and antidepressants, and in Case 2, antidepressants alone. The humiliation of such patients in a dependent role is usually overlooked. If the therapist is unaccustomed to dealing with shame (the feeling of being exposed as defective before other people) and is accustomed to dealing with fantasies involving transgression and guilt, the situation becomes more confusing. For the therapist sensitive to shame, the parts of the process that lead to reactive depression will seem obvious.

Neurotic Countertransference in the Therapist

By neurotic countertransference, I mean countertransference proper—that is, specific unresolved issues of the therapist's life transferred onto the patient or family, and not simply a reaction to the prevailing process. Such countertransferences include unresolved issues in the therapist's relationship to family members, especially parents. Prominent are feelings about their deaths, feelings of triumph over the parents, feelings of competition and greed with siblings, and so forth. Such countertransference feelings also include an intolerance of the affects so prevalent in the families of such patients: futility, depression, shame, and a host of others. For the therapist who has not acknowledged and worked out these issues, the risk of colluding with the family (often by assuming that the situation is hopeless) is extremely high.

THE CONDUCT OF THERAPY

The ultimate goals of psychotherapy are the minimization of the effects of the deficit by renegotiating family goals and the promotion of learning from experience. However, it is rare that this can be done unless the therapist has developed an empathic therapeutic process. The family is usually seen at a time when it is overwhelmed, and material resources are near exhaustion. Family members are quite likely to see the therapist's interventions as blaming them or making demands of them at a time when they cannot tolerate blame or demands.

A common sequence of effective family therapy with the patient with organic brain disease is as follows:

The Empathic Sharing of Failed Containment

This should precede the formal work-up. The therapist, when assembling the family, should discuss each member's experience in performing functions for the patient that ordinarily the patient did himself. By asking directly and tactfully whether there is agreement on the deficits, the therapist will give permission to talk about them. Often this opens communication that has been blocked by the patient's confabulation, his anger, or his catastrophic reactions. In an empathic atmosphere where the therapist as caretaker makes contact with other caretakers who are supposed to provide containment for the patient, family members are often able to talk without guilt and without blaming others to assuage the guilt. Once the therapist makes some empathic contact with each caretaker who feels helpless, exhausted, inadequate, and overburdened, much of the initial tendency of the family itself to blame and demand diminishes. If the empathic sharing of containment is bypassed, the escalation of family tensions may ensue to the point where the patient is extruded (Case Example 3). Under high tension there may be splits among caretakers—doctors fighting with doctors, wards with wards, hospitals with hospitals. When blame, demands, and shame in the family are addressed in an empathic way, these tensions have a better chance of subsiding.

While the tensions of failed containment are operative, the family may experience even history-taking as humiliating, blaming, and demanding. A full investigation of the family should be deferred until empathic contact has been made with each family member and, however briefly, with other caretaking systems, including doctors. Without such contact, inquiry itself is likely to be regarded as wounding and attacking rather than helpful.

The therapist must be able to verbalize nonjudgmentally, and to talk directly about fearful fantasies. He may, for example, ask the patient, "Do you think they'd like to be rid of you?" Or, "Do you think they're secretly dividing up your money or property, and wondering how much they get?" He may say to family members, "You may blame yourself for resenting him, or you perhaps feel what is required of you is everything you have, and that will use up all the family's resources and all of your energies and exhaust you completely." Or, "I can see how you might very well have strong feelings about not being able to rely on him in the way that you used to."

By empathizing and modeling free discussion of fantasies and fears, the therapist aids in the resolution of overwhelming anxieties and creates a forum where issues may be dealt with directly. He or she can also validate the difficulty of the caretaking task when it is no longer accompanied by companionship or sharing. What were unmentionable fantasies become anxieties to be explored openly, with at least the possibility of being minimized.

Family History

After the vulnerability to blame and demands has begun to subside, an intergenerational family history should be taken. It is important to ascertain whether a complementary set of family role assignments prior to the onset of organic brain syndrome has been disturbed in a manner that requires working through (Case Examples 1 and 2).

Reassessment

After the significance of the change in the patient is viewed in the light of the family's history, the more businesslike work of negotiation and problem-solving can begin. The actual status of the patient, both medically and psychiatrically, needs to be reassessed. Often working hypotheses concluded in an atmosphere of high tension need to be revised. Deficits can be explored within the family with great accuracy. A spouse can often tell whether the patient cannot balance a checkbook, cannot groom himself or herself, cannot find the way home, and so forth. Activities requiring foresight and planning can be assessed with extreme accuracy. These should be compared to the results of psychometric testing, and should be explained within the family setting. They form the realistic basis for later discussion of family matters, caretaking, living arrangements, and deciding exactly who is to be responsible for what. Such discussion should of course include the patient. There is a tremendous advantage if the patient's primary physician can be included in at least one such family session. A second look under circumstances of lowered emotional pressure often reveals significant diagnostic material—for example, enabling the determination of whether dementia is truly primary degenerative dementia, or subcortical, or even compounded by a large number of medications.

Medication and Management

All medications should be considered and reviewed in detail. Sedatives and minor tranquilizers, especially after a very brief time, have a disorganizing effect. Often very small doses of neuroleptics, beginning at dusk and given hourly, will avoid a "sundown" syndrome at night (Case Example 3), exacerbated by social isolation and sedatives. Antidepressant mediation or electroconvulsive therapy may be useful, and may even help with cognitive deficits due to pseudodementia but previously attributed to cerebral damage. Antidepressants must be carefully evaluated for side effects, particularly cardiovascular ones. At the same time, it is particularly important that so-called "management issues" not be split off and discussed apart from the rest of treatment and handled outside the family psychotherapy sessions. These management issues are part of the therapy, as are all containment issues, and should be discussed within the session. If they are handled somewhere else, there is a high risk that some serious containment issue will escape therapeutic scrutiny and jeopardize the whole treatment effort.

Negotiation

A realistic assessment of the family's involvement with the patient is a major area for therapeutic scrutiny. The therapist should try to make explicit whether there is agreement or disagreement about what family members think should be required of each other and of the patient. Any constriction or limitation of family members' or the patient's activities should be made fully explicit and discussed. The patient's capacity and motivation to be responsible for at least some of his actions should be explored in detail. If too much regression occurs when the patient is at home, short visits should be suggested, often at some place other than the hospital or home. A two- or three-hour meeting for dinner at a restaurant is often a great relief, both to the patient and to the family. In an enjoyable setting of this kind, regression is less likely to occur. In addition, a limited visit is often much more realistic and attractive than the prospect of spending an entire weekend with a patient who the family cannot really tolerate for longer than a few hours. The patient in turn picks up a sense that a short dinner visit is likely to be quite pleasant, as opposed to a weekend, when he or she is often resented and ignored.

Continued Support

Often the families of the OBS patient derive much benefit from multiple family groups (9) consisting of several families facing similar predicaments. Such groups provide opportunities for learning and for sharing powerful emotions—shame, guilt, anxiety, depression—with those whose situations are familiar enough to stimulate candor and genuine continuing support. Families can meet in psychotherapy groups led by a therapist or in self-help groups and organizations run largely by family members themselves. In either case, family members gain a great deal by identifying with those in similar positions—caretaker, child, spouse—and ego strength becomes additive. People gain enough support so they can learn to cope with illness and make the best possible decisions about matters they could not previously discuss.

In summary, psychotherapy is often indicated for families of patients with chronic organic brain syndrome. This psychotherapy is not simply support and reassurance but definitive working through of problems. The working through, however, is on the level of family or larger-unit systems, including all caretakers, and concerns such issues as ignorance, denial, irrational role assignments, failure of justice, retardation of maturation, intensification of pre-existing issues, blame and demands, and mis-estimate of the impact of either patient or family on each other.

The therapist involved in such treatment must have unusual skills. He or she must be able to conceptualize containment functions within entire family systems and larger caretaking systems, judging how they affect each other. For example, when an anxious family attempts to relocate a patient into a hospital, or divide caretakers so that they fight with each other, the required systems skills may be extraordinary. The therapist must also be adept at working with countertransference—that is, either the strong affects (anxiety, futility, depression) stirred up by the family situation, or neurotic countertransference enhanced by unresolved issues operative in the therapist's own family. Mastery of countertransference and the ability to work with it are crucial in any therapist who attempts to minimize dysfunctional interactive processes in a family with a member with organic brain disease and substantially alter the overall morbidity resulting from the deficit.

References

1. Pasnau R, Fawzy F, Lansky MR: Organic brain syndrome and the family, in Family Therapy and Major Psychopathology. Edited by Lansky MR. New York, Grune & Stratton, 1981

2. Shem S: The House of God. New York, Dell, 1980

3. Goldstein K: Functional disturbance in brain damage, in American Handbook of Psychiatry, vol. 1. Edited by Arieti S. New York, Basic Books, 1969

4. Lansky MR: Shame in the family relationships of borderline patients, in The Borderline Patient: Emerging Concepts in Diagnosis, Dynamics and Treatment. Edited by Grotstein J, Solomon M, Lang J. New York, Analytic Press, in press

5. Rabins PB, Mace NL, Lucas J: The impact of dementia on the family. JAMA 248:333–335, 1983

6. McAllister TW: Overview: pseudodementia. Am J Psychiatry 140:528–533, 1983

7. Lansky MR: Masks of the narcissistically vulnerable marriage. Fam Psychiatry 3:419–439, 1983

8. Bowen M: The use of family theory in clinical practice. Compr Psychiatry 7:345–374, 1966

9. Lansky MR, Bley CR, McVey GG, et al: Multiple family groups in aftercare. Int J Group Psychother 28:211–224, 1978

6

Family Therapy and Cancer: Keeping House on a Foundation of Quicksand

David K. Wellisch, Ph.D.

6

Family Therapy and Cancer: Keeping House on a Foundation of Quicksand

Families contending with cancer in a member face a wide variety of stresses. These can feel like a constant series of threats to the integrity of the family structure. One of the key underlying threats to the family is that of emotional security. At a most basic level, cancer can rob the family of any sense of continuity and predictability. Cancer can interfere with the economic stability of the family. The potential loss of the patient's ability to function occupationally combined with the loss of independence of well family members to go to work on a predictable schedule can exert a fearful grip on the family. The loss of body-image integrity is primarily experienced by the patient, but feelings about this loss often reverberate between the patient and his or her partner. Research shows that such feelings may be longer term than was previously realized (1, 2). In addition, the impending threat or actual reality of death changes the role functioning of the family members and ultimately the actual structure of the family.

The family therapist working with families bearing cancer potentially fills a multiplicity of roles. Cancer presents a wide variety of problems, dilemmas, and opportunities for change to both the family and the therapist alike. The notion that family work around cancer is limited to considerations of death and dying is unrealistic. For the family therapist to focus solely on the issues of death and dying in such families would be virtually to ignore many of the problems families bearing cancer actually face.

The purposes of this chapter are fourfold: 1) to highlight a variety of issues common in family therapy with cancer patients and their families; issues of death and dying will be included but only as a part of a larger array of clinical problems; 2) to illustrate these issues with cases I have treated; 3) to suggest some basic intervention strategies and considerations aimed partially at helping improve family-based coping with cancer, and also at optimizing change, with cancer as the impetus; and 4) to point up some key differences between family therapy in cancer-oriented situations and such therapy in noncancer situations. These differences suggest and perhaps justify changes in techniques of family therapy for families bearing cancer.

GENERAL ISSUES OF FAMILY INTERVENTION WITH CANCER

Variables That Promote Coping with Cancer

During a recent presentation to a prestigious department of surgical oncology, I sensed that the primary concern of the surgical staff from a psychological point of view was with how to predict which patient and family might "get in the most trouble" and how to head off such disasters with judicious use of their scarce psychological support personnel. The most in-depth answer to this question seemed to me to come from Project Omega, a decade-long psychological study attempting to profile "high risk" cancer patients. Their findings show that family issues, especially lack of family supportiveness and pre-illness marital dissatisfactions, are prominent but are not the only variables that characterize the high-risk group (3). Holland has conceptualized coping with cancer as depending on three highly interactive variables, one of which directly pertains to family issues. They are: 1) the premorbid level of the patient's emotional stability and lack of psychopathology, 2) the prognosis, symptoms related to the patient's disease, and difficulty in treating the patient's disease, and 3) the presence (or absence) of an emotionally supportive family matrix of the patient (4). The following case illustrates the interactive nature of these variables and their improvement in family therapy.

Case Example 1

A black woman in her 50s with metastatic breast cancer was referred by her overwhelmed oncologist for treatment of her anxiety, which verged on panic, and her (in his words) "insatiable neediness." She had been married 27 years and had two daughters, ages 19 and 23. Her husband brought her to sessions and was asked to attend the sessions, which he did with obvious interest and motivation.

By history, the patient had always been an exceedingly anxious and histrionic woman and had never coped well with stresses prior to her cancer. She had never had a satisfying relationship with her mother, as the mother constantly hovered and provoked guilt via obsessional religious ruminations and lectures. By the time she was referred, her disease was widely metastatic and not curable. The family support for her had worn thin. By the nature of her shrill, hysterical demandingness she had cowed and coerced her daughters and mother into never leaving her alone, although her husband had two jobs and was out of the house 14-16 hours daily. It was obvious that he was distancing himself and at the same time rationalizing this distancing. He repeatedly stated, "Someone has got to pay for her care." Thus, on all three of Holland's variables, this patient was sub-optimal. Her adaptation to and ability to cope with her illness were predictably poor. She held her support systems prisoner, a situation which led to dissatisfaction in everyone. Treatment consisted of pharmacologic, marital, and family intervention. She was placed on both antidepressants and minor tranquilizers (Xanax) with only minor improvements.

In the marital work, a secret emerged. The husband had had an affair out of which a child was conceived. The patient and her husband had never really worked out what this meant to them. Three things were evident: The patient lived in mortal terror of being abandoned by her husband, especially for the other woman; the patient felt jealous of the attention paid to the "other situation"; the patient felt unremitting rage and the husband profound guilt and conflict about the "other situation." Her illness thereby gave her the chance both to control him and to punish him. In the marital work he was encouraged to tell her he would not leave and that he would stay with her until her death, which was also the first time the couple had talked openly about her death. Talk of her death flowed naturally within the context of this particular marital session. In exchange for the promise on his part, she was encouraged to try to loosen her grip on him and the family. He agreed to spend more time at home, and she agreed to lessen her moment-to-moment demands.

The daughters were next brought in and encouraged to ventilate. They also felt overwhelmed and overburdened by her demands. They were given support to set limits with their mother, to negotiate her demands. It was evident that since her illness, questioning her demands had been unthinkable to them. The patient's mother, who had been brought into the home as a reserve resource, was sent home, to everyone's relief. The intensity of the situation did subside. The husband cut back his commitments to one and a half jobs and did spend more time at home. The patient made fewer demands but got more satisfying attention. The oncologist got fewer phone calls. The patient died at UCLA with the husband and daughters present several months later.

This case presents several points to consider. A crucial issue was the lengthy delay until help for the patient and family was requested by the oncologist. The family's quick acceptance of the referral probably indicated that help would have been appreciated earlier. Referring physicians sometimes need to be reminded that early referral is far more optimal in tense family situations such as this one.

As this case indicated, families with terminal cancer patients often feel too guilty and frightened of the patient's response to attempt to set necessary limits with the patient. Enabling them to do so will replace the sense of guilt with a sense of stability and frequently enable the family to give more support of better quality to the patient.

Another very important issue is the merit of combining pharmacologic, individual, and family-based therapies. This is not only appropriate but often essential. A family approach not integrated with other treatment modalities is defeating to all concerned.

This case reflects the motivation for change present in the family bearing cancer. Such motivation may derive, at first, from a sense of desperation, which stems from the factor of "family compression" recently described by Stanton (5). Stanton characterized the phenomenon as enforced involvement within a family unit, a feature which goes hand-in-glove with a chronic illness such as cancer. A secondary aspect of the motivation to change may be the family's awareness that the "clock is running out" on the present family structure. When the patient dies, no more can be done to solve interpersonal problems and relieve guilt about them. One woman recently remarked to me, "You must help me work out things with my mother *before* she dies; otherwise I will never get over my guilt about our relationship."

Primary Therapist Functions

Four functions of the therapist are paramount to me in working with families burdened by cancer. These functions are not always distinctly separate but can blend together. They involve: 1) Helping the family to negotiate with physicians and nurses. The family is constantly involved with nurses and doctors when a family member has cancer. They often live in a state of fearful dependence on these figures. They will sometimes have contradictory and ambivalent feelings about the health care deliverers, which can complicate interactions with them and lead to the patient's and the family's needs not being clearly heard or met. The family may have never before had intensive interactions with physicians and nurses and may be lost in terms of how to structure or articulate their needs. The maintenance of the relationship between the family, the patient, and the health care deliverers has profound effects on family and patient coping and adaptation to the illness (3). 2) Helping the family regain some sense of control. Facilitation of a sense of control in the context of a family member with cancer can dramatically reduce family anxiety and conflict. This involves not only enabling them to interact more effectively with the medical and nursing staff but also working with them to reinstitute at least some areas of familiarity and predictability in their daily lives. 3) Facilitating interaction and communication within the family. Often when cancer is diagnosed in a family member the family unit deteriorates into a set of individuals who are so dedicated to protecting each other's feelings, especially the patient's, that communication ceases—and along with it mutual support. The facilitation of family communication reduces isolation, increases support, and promotes mutual decision-making, which is very necessary in dealing with cancer. As in family therapy with all other problems, facilitation of communication is the bedrock for family-based coping with cancer. 4) Facilitating grief, when appropriate, within the family. Grief may be present at many stages of the family's experience with cancer. The periods of diagnosis, recurrence of disease, terminality, and postdeath are classically associated with grief for the patient and the family. At all of these points the family interaction may be constricted or paralyzed with unexpressed or unresolved grief. In addition, parents serve as powerful models for children in expressing grief. Intervention, even in one sector of the family (such as the parents), may have profound consequences for another sector of the family (such as the children) even if that sector is never seen in consultation or treatment.

Four cases will be discussed to illustrate these points. Case Example 2 illustrates the way in which a therapist can help family members to negotiate with health care providers.

Case Example 2

John, the adult son of a man in his 70s with a metastatic and terminal brain tumor, came for family consultation with his wife, Sarah. John had brought his father and mother to the West Coast for further evaluation and possible treatment after his father's brain surgery. The evaluation had been done and the father was undergoing daily radiation therapy at the time the younger couple consulted me. They were grief-stricken. Neither John nor Sarah had previously experienced a major illness in a family member. They had never talked to doctors in any depth and had little confidence in doing so at present. They observed that the father was more and more exhausted as the eight-week course of radiation unfolded. They began to doubt that the radiation treatment was worth the effort for the father. The father, left partially aphasic by the brain surgery, struggled to say, "I want to go home," midway through the course of radiation. The couple could not seem to get a satisfactory answer from the oncologist about whether finishing the radiation would realistically extend the father's life or enhance the quality of the time that remained. The couple brought John's mother to the family sessions. She wanted to go home and supported her husband's statements that he wanted to go home. I recommended that the family obtain a second opinion on their oncologic questions, which they did. The consultant felt that the radiation could in no way guarantee help to the father. I talked directly to the first oncologist and urged him to talk with the family in greater depth about their concerns. He was shocked that they had talked with me so pointedly about these issues. "They should have been talking to me," he stated. I agreed. He arranged a meeting with the entire family, at which it was agreed that the patient and his wife would return to the East Coast and resume care, decidedly palliative and only for symptom relief, from their family doctor.

This case illustrates the family's need for support and clarification in dealing directly with health care personnel. Sometimes, direct contact between a family therapist (mental health professional) and medical health care deliverers is essential in facilitating such direct communication. This does *not* mean that the family therapist talks *for* the family but does mean the therapist attempts to set or clarify an agenda for discussion between the parties. Often the medical personnel will listen more closely if the therapist formulates the problem in a manner that calms anxieties about direct discussion.

The following three cases address the issue of facilitation of communication and grief.

Case Example 3

A man with a wife and three children (ages 7, 11, and 14) died of melanoma, after a 30-month illness. I saw this couple, and the patient alone, often during his decline. He was a powerful and intellectually brilliant man who endured his illness with the stoicism that had characterized his life. One interaction I observed between the patient and his wife seemed to characterize his coping, as well as his expectations of how his wife and family should cope with his illness and death. As she sat on his hospital bed and began to cry, he pushed his hand forcefully on top of hers and said, "Be strong dear, be strong." The pushing down of his hand seemed also to command her to push down her grief and tears. In visits alone, the patient fretted over not having bought more life insurance and about whether his wife would be able to carry on his ethical traditions and academic expectations with the children. The element of pure grief never surfaced in him in an emotional way. After the patient died, the youngest son began to experience episodes of a kind of derealization. This exceedingly bright 7-year-old said to me after one of these, "My mother seemed like a robot to me; I thought the real mother was down in the basement."

This statement not only showed me the serious upset of the child but also struck me as being a guarded but accurate observation of the mother. When we arranged for the boy to see a child psychiatrist by himself, the psychiatrist confirmed that the continuation of family-based therapy was of primary importance for the boy and for his family. Taking the boy's symbolic statement literally presented a mandate and blueprint for the therapy. The task became to give the mother confidence to show her true self. She had feared that showing the children her grief would be disloyal to her dead husband's wishes and would upset the children even more. She gradually became able to express her grief more openly. She returned for consultation three years later stating, "The kids are too rigid; none of us have worked through our grief enough yet."

Case Example 4

A couple in their 30s came for therapy shortly after the husband's diagnosis of Hodgkin's Disease. Their immediate concerns included how his diagnosis would affect their marriage and how his diagnosis and treatment would affect their two boys, ages 2½ and 4. Communication appeared difficult for this couple, and they indicated having difficulties talking about his illness with each other was well as with their older boy. The couple felt stuck as to how to proceed to talk with the older boy, who seemed to want to know what was wrong with his father. I asked them to bring the older boy in, and in our session together I asked him to draw a family picture. He drew his father's face with a big smile and with golden dots around the eyes. When asked about his father's face the boy explained, "My father is smiling on the outside, but crying on the inside."

Shortly after this session the couple reported that the family pet bird died. While the father buried it in the backyard, the boy spontaneously said to his mother, "If Daddy dies, will you just marry another Daddy in a few days?" Following these two incidents, the couple agreed that talking with the child about the basic details of his father's illness was indicated, given that the boy intuited with impressive accuracy the emotional issues related to the illness. It was apparent to the couple that the boy did not need to be protected from such information and that he was not fragile psychologically in this area. This served as the opening phase of the therapy, as the couple indicated no further difficulties in talking with their older son. The communication problem with the child appeared to serve as a catalyst for working on the couple's hesitancy to talk with each other both about the husband's illness and about other marital stresses.

Case Example 5

A 34-year-old woman was seen with her husband and her son after her diagnosis of metastatic melanoma. The couple had been married 14 years and had a 12-year-old son. I had seen this family previously for the son's problems with school and weight. In the previous course of therapy the son and mother had seemed intensely over-involved, with the husband remaining in a more distant and peripheral position in the family. Some progress had been made on this prior to her cancer diagnosis, with the son and father becoming somewhat more involved and the son becoming more independent from his mother. After her diagnosis, the family was seen sporadically, as she was treated with very debilitating chemotherapy that kept her homebound. It has also been my experience that families living with cancer will not consistently remain in family therapy but, rather, come as a family when a crisis develops for them.

Such a crisis was evident when the patient was dying. At this point, her two best friends called me, insisting that we have a session including her husband, the son, and the two friends. In the session the source of the two friends' concerns was readily evident. It soon became clear that the son was not being prepared to deal with the reality of his mother's medical situation. The son did not know the name of his mother's disease (neither "cancer" nor "melanoma"). He also did not know she was terminally ill or that she would soon die. (Her death occurred within two weeks of this session.) The friends were enraged at the husband, who was obviously emotionally paralyzed and unable to talk with his son about his mother's true condition. Just prior to the session, I had talked at length with the mother's oncologist, who urged me to discuss frankly the patient's situation. He offered to see the son and the father the next day if they wished. During our session, the name of the mother's condition was given and her terminality was described, but no time frame was offered as the oncologist was hesitant to commit to that. The son was tearful but not overwhelmed. The father was clearly overwhelmed. In his grief, the father revealed his own father's early demise and the absence of anyone to help him with his feelings at that time. The father appeared to over-identify with his son, and in doing so had not been able to communicate with nor offer emotional support to the boy. The two friends were also intensely involved in the session. The father had previously resented their

> involvement, but now seemed to see their presence as supportive. The friends saw the father differently in the process of the session. Previously they had viewed him as deliberately interfering with his son's access to information about his mother. In the session we all saw the father's almost inconsolable grief at this second major loss, which he was attempting to deny. His denial had reinforced his son's denial. Once this impasse was broken, the father saw that the son could cope and he himself also coped. The friends were very supportive to the son after that, and the father accepted their support and involvement.

Several points from Case Examples 3, 4, and 5 warrant discussion. Common to all three of these cases is the emergence of grief when communication is facilitated by the family therapist. As was evident in Case Examples 3 and 5, the adults may defend against the expression of their grief by projection of their own feelings of vulnerability onto their children. This protects the adults, not the children. The children, as all three of the cases reflect, may be ready earlier than the adults to grapple with the grief and feelings generated by the cancer.

A second important issue demonstrated by Case Examples 3 and 5 is the sequence of work possible for families burdened with cancer. They may come for family sessions sporadically and episodically during the patient's illness. They also may not be able to work through or face powerful feelings until late in the illness, or until years after a death, as illustrated by Case 3. In my experience, such families may need to come and go, and this does not represent therapeutic failure. The pattern is so common with such families that I cannot usefully see it as resistance. I have come to see it as the pace by which family therapy is possible when cancer is the impetus.

Case Examples 3 and 5 underscore the fact that legacies of past losses impact on the current family interaction and can affect coping. Reilly has brilliantly described this theme for families with suicidally drug-abusing offspring (6). The influence of past losses also affects therapists treating these families. Countertransference feelings in the therapist in regard to resolution of his or her past losses must be carefully considered. Failure to consider such countertransference can lead to therapeutic errors, usually not impeding the family's progress but rather pushing them to go faster than they are able.

In Case Example 3, the legacy was the dead husband's verbal and nonverbal commandment on how to live after his death. His inability to react to his terminality emotionally made it impossible for his family to premourn prior to his death. Mourning after his death meant disobeying him. This was emotionally experienced by the family as a cause for guilt, representing a disconnection with his values and style, which they had needed to see as functional. The recognition that his style might not have been the most functional for them led to confusion and to anger about him, which further complicated the mourning process. In Case Example 5, the father's unresolved grief reaction served to further complicate his own son's already difficult but *not* impossible task. The father had not been able to utilize the friends in the current situation because he had been unable to see the difference between the present situation and that of his past, where there were no friends to help.

IMPACT OF CANCER ON MARITAL PROCESSES

In this section, the focus on the marital relationships within the family structure will have two parts. In the first part, some predictable effects of cancer on the marital relationship will be discussed, with cases to illustrate these effects. In the second part, types of pathological marriages will be discussed as they are uniquely affected by cancer, again with illustrative cases.

Marital Functions

The impact of cancer on the marital relationship is multifaceted—a complicated equation that includes the ability of the individual partners to withstand stress and frustration, the history of the relationship, and all of the disease and treatment factors of the patient. Three key issues will be particularly focused upon here. In my experience they are universal issues in marriage that are always affected by the presence and pressures of cancer and its treatment.

The first factor is the couple's experience with the changes in their dependence and independence, as affected by the cancer. Often the pattern is that the ill partner becomes more situationally, physically, and emotionally dependent on the well partner. Conversely, the well partner finds himself or herself faced with a loss of independence. Sometimes this picture can be reversed, with the well partner becoming so frightened by the diagnosis or course of the illness that he or she becomes overdependent on the ill partner. The pre-illness balance of dependence-independence in the relationship is always changed by the cancer. In the early stages of the illness or during a time of minimal treatment such a change can be minimal. In the later stages of an illness or in the midst of intensive treatment, this shift can radically alter the interaction in the relationship.

A second important factor is the couple's experience with intimacy and communication, as affected by the cancer. Following the changes in dependence and loss of independence, the couple find themselves placed in an emotional context with each other of powerfully heightened feelings, fears, and pressures. Often the ill partner has dramatically heightened needs to be supported, to talk, and especially to be heard and understood by the well partner. The well partner often feels the conflict of genuinely wanting to be supportive and understanding but also feeling very stressed and burdened by the partner's increased needs. Not uncommonly, the well partner also has heightened needs for support but has no one to offer such support. Cancer presents many decisions to be made by the couple, ranging from minimal to matters of life and death. Problems in communication of emotional issues usually also means problems in decision-making.

A third factor that can be affected by the cancer is the couple's sexual relationship. Most couples experience temporary effects in this area, especially right after surgery or during chemotherapy or radiation, which are quickly resolved. A minority of couples describe their sexual relations as better after cancer. This may be due to the enormous emotional impact cancer presents, which creates a major motivation to reappraise the bond between the partners. A minority of couples describe a major deterioration in their sexual relations after cancer. This may be due, in part, to physical sequalae of disease and treatment. Experience has shown me, however, that it is equally as likely to result from a combination of emotional, communicational, role-change, and physical factors. Two cases will illustrate these issues and their interaction in the cancer-burdened couple.

Case Example 6

A couple sought help with me for marital dysfunction subsequent to the earlier diagnosis of the wife's breast cancer, now metastatic. Their marriage, dysfunctional prior to her diagnosis, was now severely stressed. She was very ill, but sex was still possible for the couple. Nevertheless, they had not had sex for several months. It emerged that this couple had previously kept a generous degree of distance between them, both situationally and emotionally. Now they were unable to keep this distance. The cancer forced them to spend more time together and forced them to communicate more than ever before. The patient was forced to depend on her husband, an abrupt role reversal from prior times in their marriage. On the husband's part, he severely missed his former freedom to spend large amounts of time outside the house. He felt exceedingly guilty about the wish to be away from her. He communicated very little to his wife except agitation and discomfort, which increased her depression and her sense of feeling like a burden to him.

Intervention took place on several levels. First, the couple were encouraged to ventilate their frustrations. Both learned that the other felt the same: trapped, resentful, frightened. Second, the couple were encouraged to regain some of the distance they had needed previously. This required some help from friends. It also required the patient to give her husband permission to go out. Third, the couple were *not* encouraged to resume sex immediately. Rather, they were encouraged to try to reassume husband-wife roles in an attempt to push back the father-daughter roles imposed by the illness. This took the form, for example, of having him take her out to dinner when possible. The couple were not effectively able to resume an active sexual life, as she ultimately became terminally ill and physically quite wasted. At this point, the therapy became less maritally oriented and more individually based with each of the spouses. At the time of this writing she remains alive but critically ill.

In our research on problems of home-bound cancer patients, we found data in a large population which substantiated the severe problems that younger couples (those under 50) have with role shifts, that leave one spouse very dependent on the other, as reflected in Case Example 6. This was in bold contrast to older couples (50 or more), where such shifts were not as significant a problem (7).

Case Example 7

A couple in their 50s saw me for increased marital tension, which had intensified after the wife's breast cancer and mastectomy. The husband was a very successful professional man. The wife had been a busy homemaker and mother of two children, the last of whom had left the house subsequent to her mastectomy. She described their marriage as one where she typically listened at great lengths to him about business. He, however, was not accustomed to listening to her problems. Now she had a far greater need to talk and be heard than ever before. He was abrupt with her, unable to listen effectively to her feelings about her disease and surgery. She had become sexually less available to him, a pattern she identified as stemming from "being turned-off by his insensitivity to me." The couple became increasingly irritated with each other, and a new and upsetting pattern emerged in their interactions. He began to listen even less and angrily accused her of not caring about his feelings. She began to withdraw further, becoming less sexually available and less emotionally giving, for the first time, she contemplated separation.

As the marital therapy unfolded, several things became evident. First, he had lost his mother as a child. He was very reluctant to face and listen to her feelings about her cancer, which seemed to reintroduce to him his unresolved mourning about the loss of his mother. He related feeling "helpless then and feeling helpless now." He indicated that when his wife spoke of her feelings and became upset, he was at a total loss as to how to make her feel better.

The therapy focused heavily on these issues. The husband was encouraged to see his wife's cancer as having an excellent prognosis, unlike his mother's illness. This helped him to begin to separate the two situations in his mind. He was emotionally very unprepared to resolve his grief about his mother but was prepared to rethink the notion that he had to make his wife feel better when she cried or verbalized painful feelings about her illness. It was evident that he attempted to suppress her in order to repress his own feelings. Initially, he had difficulties accepting the notion that just listening to her in a supportive way and not trying to make her feel different was a helpful thing to do. This seemed rather passive and ineffectual for this very action-oriented businessman. However, he did try this approach and liked the fact that she again seemed interested in him. He was puzzled by the idea that being a listener (passive in his thinking) was really being active and helpful. She was strongly encouraged to view his behavior a bit more empathically in the light of his early loss, and to recognize how this affected their current relationship difficulties. Initially, she was so angry at him that she rejected this possibility, but gradually she became willing to look more deeply at why he could not seem to support her more satisfactorily. The couple dealt with her breast reconstruction more successfully than they had dealt with her mastectomy. They attended the presurgical consultations together, and he spent more time listening to her feelings about the reconstruction.

These two cases reflect sharp differences yet share similarities. Although both patients were diagnosed with the same illness, one has a good prognosis while the other will die. Even in the light of these completely different clinical courses, their marriages experienced similar pressures. Both couples experienced radical shifts in the level of dependency of one spouse upon another. Both couples needed to talk about the new feelings, pressures, and concerns produced by the cancer, yet both couples lacked the communication skills to do so when necessary. Both couples were faced with the effects of these emotional and communication difficulties on their sexual relations. Even though the outcomes of the illness are radically different, the effects on the marital relationship can be remarkably similar.

Pathological Marriages in the Cancer Context

Many cancer patients are blessed with the security and protection of a stable, flexible, and supportive marriage, which undeniably helps them better adapt to and cope with their illness (8, 9). Unfortunately, this is not universally the case. We have seen several unstable marriages falter or become much more unstable due to cancer, its treatment, and its outcome. Marital conflict has a demonstrably negative effect on adaptation to cancer (3). I will discuss three types of pathological marital interactional patterns:

1) the avoider-pursuer marriage, 2) the "doll house" marriage, and 3) the alcoholic marriage.

Case Example 8: An Avoider-Pursuer Marriage

The patient, a man of 49, was seen in the hospital on an emergency consultation because of suicidal ideation which alarmed the hospital staff nurses and his attending physician. He had metastatic melanoma and had been hospitalized for chemotherapy. The suicidal crisis was precipitated by his finding out, while hospitalized, that his wife was having an affair. He hired a private detective to follow his wife, and the report on her activities was brought to him in the hospital. His suicidal feelings were abated temporarily with focused support and medication. The patient's wife was then interviewed separately. She detailed a lengthy marital history of his over-involvement with business and also with other women. She was quick to clarify, "I don't think his other love is women; it has always been his business, that is his real mistress." She refused marital therapy and indicated an intention to persist in her extramarital relationship. It became clear that she was angry at him and felt so rejected by him that now his cancer made no real difference to her. She remarked, "Just because he needs me now does not mean that I will now be there. He was never there for me."

The patient was not pleased by his wife's perception of their marriage but could not disagree. The couple decided to separate and not divorce. He was provided with support by the ward nurses and began to participate in individual supportive therapy. His daughter, a woman in her 20s who worked for him, became his business partner and took over the business after his death.

This case presented some complicated therapeutic questions. First, did we have to delve at all into his family issues? His oncologist requested only that we respond to the patient's suicidal distress. It seemed to us that trying to reduce his distress without family intervention was like putting towels in front of a bathroom door to stem a flood from an overflowing bathtub. To continue the metaphor, we chose to go in and turn off the faucets of the bathtub. Second, we wondered whether or not to try to patch up the marriage until his death. Experience with other couples has shown us this is unwise—that support of such an overtly hostile spouse is not useful. Rather, we chose to set up dependable support from outside the marriage. Since this placed more of a burden on the staff, we then worked on carefully defining the limits of their ability to support and nurture him. We worked on the staff's understanding of the dynamics of this marriage so that they could grasp how the wife could deny the husband support at this point in his illness. It was particularly important to clarify the "avoider-pursuer pattern" as one in which this couple chronically exchanged these roles. It was necessary for the staff to know that he, too, had previously been unfaithful. They came to see that this behavior pattern regulated the little intimacy possible between these partners yet maintained a sense of challenge and excitement in the marriage. It was initially easy for the staff to characterize the wife as the worst form of villain rather than seeing the marriage as previously stabilized by the avoider-pursuer transactions, which could no longer be tolerated in the light of his cancer. It was all too easy to see him as utterly victimized in his current circumstances.

The next case exemplifies aspects of a marital syndrome earlier characterized by Pittman and Flomenhoft as (taking their cue from Ibsen) "The Doll's House Marriage" (10). In this marital interaction one spouse (often the male partner, but not always) cannot tolerate acknowledgment of the other partner's competence. The doll partner, although protesting otherwise, is often profoundly invested in the role, which offers security and dependency-need gratification at the price of surrendering one's competence. Such marriages achieve a pathologically stable equilibrium but are obviously prone to crisis from external events that assault this equilibrium. Cancer in a partner, especially the "master," is just such a disequilibrium-inducing crisis.

Case Example 9: A Doll's House Marriage

In one couple that sought marital therapy, the man had metastatic lung cancer with a poor prognosis. His wife, he complained, spent her days shopping and would not take measures to "grow up, pitch in, and really help me." As their marriage was further discussed, it became evident that he viewed her as an attractive ornament ("a real doll") rather than a person to be taken seriously. When she attempted to take

> steps toward setting limits with one of their children, he was not supportive in backing her as an equal with authority. He was not prepared to give up control to her in any area. He updated his will and provided for his wife and three children simply as though he had four children. She was not included in the deliberations with his attorney. The therapy focused on his overfunctioning, with two goals: 1) that he step out of her way so that she could assume responsibility, and 2) that she stop subtly influencing him to take control when she felt threatened, anxious, or uncertain. She accepted the suggestion of individual therapy to modify this pattern, realizing that his terminal illness and subsequent death would give her no choice but to take responsibility for her life. She became quite determined to prepare herself for managing her life after his demise.

This case reflects, as do the others in this section, a long-standing marital syndrome generated by the mutual interlocking pathology of the partners (11). The presence of cancer in a spouse does not usually ameliorate these patterns, as Case Example 9 indicates. However, the presence of cancer may present an impetus for change, as is also evidenced in Case 9. In a surprising number of such situations I have seen this impetus for change motivate the couple to modify their costly and pathological symbiosis. Clinical intervention, even if unsuccessful previously, may be more likely to succeed when cancer is in the picture and it is ominously apparent that change is inevitable. Thus, resistance in work with cancer-burdened families may actually be less of a limiting factor than it would be with the same family or couple in therapy prior to the diagnosis of cancer. The underlying motivation comes from several varieties of fear, especially fear of loss of control, abandonment, mutilation, or pain.

The next case will underscore the capacity for change in a marital or family structure burdened with cancer even when monumental pathology and resistance is present. This case involves many elements, including alcoholism in a spouse.

Alcoholism involves at least nine million adults and their families, so it is no surprise that alcoholism becomes a serious issue in many families with cancer. In confronting such a marital or family unit, it has been useful for me to consider carefully at least three key points presented by Berenson in his conceptualization of alcoholism and the family system: 1) The alcoholic (parent) in the family system periodically becomes symptomatic as an *adaptive* or *stabilizing* mechanism for the family system, 2) both spouses feel powerless in their attempts to control each other and are often involved in futile, escalating attempts to gain power and control, and 3) if and when the "dry" spouse stops trying to make the "wet" spouse stop drinking, the likelihood that the "wet" spouse will stop increases dramatically (12).

Case Example 10: An Alcoholic Marriage

In a couple in their 40s who came for marital therapy, the wife had a life-threatening metastatic head and neck cancer. They had three children, a girl in her early 20s, a girl in her late teens, and a boy in his mid-teens. The first marital session was illustrative of what was to follow as her illness progressed and her condition deteriorated. In this session the obviously dying, frail-looking woman immediately set the agenda in a blunt fashion. She stated, "I'm upset about dying, but I'm most upset about the thought of leaving my kids at the mercy of my husband's drunken behavior." The husband, a large, nattily dressed man, responded, "I am not an alcoholic," and then launched into a series of self-justifying statements such as, "I never drink in the morning," "I have never lost a day's work due to drinking," "My health is excellent. Now could an alcoholic be as healthy as I am?"

A struggle for control was evident in this couple. One current goal of hers was to ensure funds for the children that he could not withdraw after episodes of anger at them. Their marital history included episodes of his not coming home at night, having arrests for driving while intoxicated, and having affairs. It was evident that the classic alcoholic marital roles in errant son and controlling mother were well represented in this couple.

In later sessions the children were seen conjointly with the parents and were also seen as a separate subsystem of the family. The children presented a paradox. They were clearly in a close alliance with the mother but reflected little grief about her terminality, of which they were as knowledgeable as the parents. In the family context, the father appeared distanced from the family and alone. His position seemed to exemplify that described by Jackson in her classic paper on the adjustment of the family to alcoholism, where the "wet" spouse (usually father and husband) is eased outside the family routine and essentially has no role inside the family (13). The middle daughter seemed closest to her mother and most identified with her in terms of assuming her functions and running the household. The older daughter and younger son seemed less central.

In one phase of the therapy the father asked for an individual session. He related painful guilt over his affairs and pain in his feelings of alienation from his children. He emphasized a long-standing pattern of seeing his wife as a madonna-like figure whom he could revere but not relate to sexually. This function, he felt, could only be fulfilled with a series of extramarital liaisons. In the context of the individual session he seemed to feel less defensive about exploring his drinking. It was evident that the idea that his drinking might make a reconciliation impossible with his children after his wife's death was very disturbing to him. My reinforcement of this possibility led him to ask for help with his drinking. He was referred to both a physician who specialized in medical care of alcohol-related problems and to AA. He attended and saw the physician. He did have a few binges as his wife became sicker, and was arrested for "driving under the influence" on one of these occasions.

The most dramatic family conflict occurred at a point when the patient clearly was too ill to cope alone in the home and help was needed on a continual basis. The husband adamantly refused to allow help into the home. He indicated, "My daughters can take over those functions. Why do we need strangers in the house? The house is too small." The oncologist and I joined to support the wife on this issue. It seemed evident that the husband was attempting to shift his subtle but intense dependency from his wife onto his daughters, especially the younger one. Previously, his disapproval of his younger daughter's boyfriend had kept her from individuating from the family. His wife had identified his disapproval as a form of pathological control.

The issue of the household help became a turning point in the therapy and in the husband's adjustment. He did accept help in the home and in doing so seemed to accept his children's need to individuate and lead separate lives. The children saw this and became more supportive and interested in him. Family grief became more evident; they were now really preparing for their wife and mother to die. During the final period the father became earnestly involved in AA and was quite supportive of his wife.

The family returned for a follow-up a year after the patient's death. The children were still living with the father; neither of the daughters had chosen to go away to school. They both were dating, however, and the father was not interfering or critical of their choices. In addition, he proudly related, "I am not now drinking at all."

This case illustrates several points. First, we did not make cessation of the man's drinking a central or exclusive goal. Support of the patient in her dying became central. The husband felt even more left behind and felt that this was his last chance to re-enter the family. He had to give to get back into the family and chose to do so by beginning to work toward sobriety. If stopping his drinking was chosen as the only goal, it probably would only have aggravated the chronic power struggle in this family. The dying patient's needs were fully supported by the oncologist and myself. Our alliance overwhelmed the husband's resistance and pathological needs to make his daughter into a combination pseudo-spouse and nurse/housekeeper. I have written previously about the danger of an adolescent's being converted into this role when a parent has cancer (14). The binges of the husband were momentarily adaptive in a paradoxical way for the family, in that they diverted attention from the hopeless problem of the patient's dying toward a problem with some promise of alleviation. The binges also brought attention to the husband's needs, albeit in a pathological fashion. He learned in the therapy that he did not have to have the binges in order to receive attention for his needs.

As with the previous case, the terminal cancer of this woman did two positive things. It made a family available for therapy that would previously have not been available. It also forced the wife to stop trying to control the husband. Instead it placed the pressure squarely on him to decide if he wanted to re-enter the family by changing his behavior. Resistance was not absent in this case but was much more easily managed than would have been possible at almost any other time in the family history.

THE DYNAMICS OF UNORTHODOX CANCER TREATMENTS AND THE FAMILY

The lure of unorthodox cancer treatments is a phenomenon that poses a dilemma for almost all cancer patients and their families. The reasons underlying pursuit of unorthodox treatment are both interesting and pathetic. Holland has summarized several reasons why patients and their families may seek such unproven remedies: 1) A search for a second opinion or reason for error in the diagnosis; 2) the wish to counteract a sense of hopelessness and helplessness about the prospect of facing uncontrollable disease, or reasserting personal control; 3) the wish in patients and families to find an instant "cure" which has no adverse side effects (15). In addition, the guilt of the family can lead them to try anything rather than feel they have given up.

Several beliefs about patients and families who seek unorthodox cancer treatments were found to be untrue in a study of 660 cancer patients, of whom 282 had only conventional therapy, 325 had conventional and unorthodox therapy, and 53 had only unorthodox therapy. First, patients who sought unorthodox treatment were better educated, included a larger percentage of Caucasians, and enjoyed more family support than those who sought conventional treatment alone. Second, the percentage of patients who sought unorthodox treatment early in their clinical course was almost identical to the number who sought it late in their course (terminal or end-stage). Third, the practitioners whom these patients sought for unorthodox treatments were as likely to be licensed physicians as anything else (16).

The conflictual attractions of unorthodox treatments have led to some of the most complex, painful, and challenging clinical interactions that I have seen in my work with families burdened with cancer. Two cases will illustrate a few of these issues.

Case Example 11

A middle-aged couple came for marital therapy because of the pressures imposed by the wife's metastatic lung cancer. Both partners agreed that the marriage had been conflictual and difficult for years. He complained that she was "hysterical and demanding"; she complained that he was "unaffectionate, cold." At one point in the therapy he started pushing her very hard to consider unorthodox treatment. In a self-conscious, almost apologetic fashion, this high-level business executive described a program he had found in Mexico where patients were "purified of toxins and kept on diets of fresh fruits and juices." He suggested that rather than going on a planned vacation they go to this program instead. She responded, "I've had enough doctors. I need a vacation a lot more than I need another program." He heard this as a definitive "No" and stopped pushing her. Shortly afterward he asked for an individual session. He was heavily burdened with guilt and explained that he had recently entered into a relationship with another woman after feeling imprisoned and deprived by his wife's lengthy illness. He felt terribly guilty about proceeding with the relationship but did not want to end it as it was meeting some of his needs. The correlation between his starting the affair and pushing the unconventional therapy on his wife was pointed out. He saw this association immediately and remarked, "I guess I tried to make up for my feelings of guilt for abandoning her by giving her something extra whether she needed it or not." The patient died without further pressure of this sort by her husband.

Case Example 12

The dynamics in this case are the reverse of those in the previous case. Here, the patient, a woman in her 50s, had lung cancer and was demanding that her family take her to Tijuana, Mexico, for unorthodox treatment. Her demand was made late in her illness and was presented with the threat, "If you don't do this for me, you will all feel guilty after I die that you did not give me what I needed." The family acceded to her wishes and did take her to Mexico shortly before her death, despite concerns voiced by her oncologist. In my consultation with the family and oncologist, I made two recommendations. I recommended to the oncologist that he leave the door open to the patient even though he vigorously disagreed with what she was doing. I encouraged him to view her decision to go to Mexico not as a sign that he had failed but rather as an example of predictable behavior in this woman. She had a powerful need for control, which was being expressed around her terminality, where she felt a profound loss of control. He accepted my recommendation, and their relationship was maintained. I recommended to the family that they cooperate, however reluctantly, with her request, but on one condition—that she would agree to go to only one treatment center in Mexico. I have seen patients and families get on a merry-go-round at this point which takes them from clinic to clinic, city to city, and even continent to continent. The patient did agree to this condition, eventually returned to the care of her oncologist, and died in Los Angeles.

As these two cases illustrate, the pressure for unorthodox treatments can come from the family, the patient, and, in some instances, both. The family therapist is well advised, as in Case

Example 11, to look carefully for subtle dynamics which promote the urging of unorthodox treatment.

Case Example 12 reflects the need by both the family and treatment system for the family therapist to be a negotiator, limit setter, and clarifier for both groups (family and treaters). Perhaps most important of all, as reflected in Case Example 12, is the direct role of the family therapist in the maintenance of the relationship between the oncologist, patient, and family. Rarely does this relationship become more threatened than when the specter of unorthodox therapy is raised.

SUMMARY

This chapter reflects the multiplicity of roles performed by the family therapist who works with cancer-burdened families. As demonstrated by the complexity of the 12 cases described, the notion that family work around cancer is limited to considerations of death and dying is illusory. Family therapy certainly can and must, when appropriate, focus on grief, death, and dying. However, as these cases show, the possibilities for change are very rich in this context. The family therapist can "seize the moment" and facilitate growth in the family as well as ways of adapting to and coping with the cancer. To focus only on the cancer is to minimize the potential provided by this unique event in the family history. Paradoxical as it may seem, the cancer is both a catastrophe and an opportunity for the family if the therapy provides appropriate guidance.

References

1. Maguire GP, Lee EG, Bevington DJ, et al: Psychiatric problems in the first year after mastectomy. Br Med J 281:963–965, 1978

2. Maguire GP, Tait A, Brooke M: Psychiatric morbidity and physical toxicity associated with chemotherapy after mastectomy. Br Med J 281:1179–1180, 1980

3. Weisman AD, Worden JW, Sobel HJ: Psychosocial screening and intervention with cancer patients: research report. Project Omega, Department of Psychiatry, Harvard Medical School, Massachusetts General Hospital, 1980

4. Holland J: Humanistic side of cancer care: impact and implications for patients. Presented at Fifth Annual Cancer Symposium, Scripps Memorial Hospital, San Diego, 1981

5. Stanton MD: Fusion, compression, diversion and the workings of paradox: a theory of therapeutic systemic change. Fam Process 23:135–169, 1984

6. Reilly, DM: Family factors in the etiology and treatment of youthful drug abuse. Fam Ther 2:149–171, 1975

7. Wellisch DK, Fawzy FI, Landsverk J, et al: Evaluation of psychosocial problems of the home-bound cancer patient: the relationship of disease and the sociodemographic variables of patients to family problems. J Psychosoc Onc 1:1–15, 1983

8. Funch DP, Marshall S: The role of stress, social support and age in survival from breast cancer. J Psychosom Res 27:77–83, 1983

9. Vachon MLS: The importance of social support in the longitudinal adaptation to bereavement and breast cancer. Presented at the annual American Psychological Association Meeting, New York, 1979

10. Pittman FS, Flomenhoft K: Treating the doll's house marriage. Fam Process 9:143–155, 1970

11. Ackerman NW: Family pyschotherapy and psychoanalysis: implications of difference. Fam Process 1:30–43, 1962

12. Berenson D: Alcohol and the family system, in Family Therapy: Theory and Practice. Edited by Guerin P. New York, Gardiner Press, 1977

13. Jackson JK: The adjustment of the family to the crisis of alcoholism. Q J Stud Alcohol 15:562–586, 1954

14. Wellisch D: Adolescent acting out when a parent has cancer. Int J Fam Ther 1:230–241, 1979

15. Holland S: Why patients seek unproven cancer remedies: a psychological perspective. Journal for Clinicians 32:10–14, 1982

16. Cassileth BA, Lusk EJ, Strouse TB, et al: Contemporary unorthodox treatments in cancer medicine. Ann Int Med 101:105–112, 1984